PREVENTING
HEART DISEASE

PREVENTING
HEART DISEASE

The Coronary Prevention Group

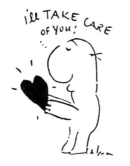

i'll TAKE CARE
OF YOU!

BOOKS

Published by Consumers' Association
and Hodder & Stoughton

Which? Books are commissioned by
The Association for Consumer Research
and published by Consumers' Association
2 Marylebone Road, London NW1 4DX and
Hodder & Stoughton, 47 Bedford Square, London WC1B 3DP
Preventing Heart Disease was researched by the
Coronary Prevention Group
and written by Jeanette Longfield of the
Coronary Prevention Group

Typographic design by Paul Saunders
Cover design by Ivor Claydon
Cover photographs by courtesy of The Image Bank and
Sally and Richard Greenhill
Cartoons by 'Larry'

First edition June 1991
Copyright © 1991 Consumers' Association Ltd

British Library Cataloguing in Publication Data
Preventing heart disease.
  1. Humans. Heart. Diseases. Prevention
  I. Longfield, Jeanette   II. Consumers' Association
  616.1205

ISBN 0 340 53900 3

Typeset by Litho Link Limited, Welshpool, Powys
Printed and bound in Great Britain by BPCC Hazell Books,
Aylesbury, Bucks. Member of BPCC Limited

CONTENTS

THE CORONARY PREVENTION GROUP

EVERYBODY has to die from something in the end and people often say that a heart attack is a quick and easy way to go. But, as this book shows, coronary heart disease kills many people long before their time: one man in 12 dies of it before the age of 65. Countless thousands suffer the disabling pain of angina.

Coronary heart disease is the leading cause of death in the UK, claiming over 170,000 lives every year. Apart from the impact on sufferers, their families and friends, coronary heart disease costs the country a fortune – nearly £2 billion a year in lost earnings, or 40 million working days (that's over ten times the number lost by strikes). Treating coronary heart disease costs the NHS over £500 million a year – but only £10 million is spent on preventing it.

The Coronary Prevention Group is the only UK charity dedicated to the prevention of coronary heart disease. We aim to cut coronary deaths by 30 per cent by the year 2000 – that's 1,000 lives saved every week – and we need your help to do it.

If you would like to support our work, please write to the address below for details of how you can help. We won't swamp you with junk mail and we won't pass your name on to any other organisation. We will send you our magazine *Heart*, a free copy of new booklets, and an annual report on what we achieve with your money – and our heartfelt thanks.

The Coronary Prevention Group
102 Gloucester Place
London W1H 3DA

FOREWORD

HEART disease kills one in four people in the United Kingdom. Many of these deaths can be prevented if people make healthy choices about their lifestyle. People will make healthy choices if they have the relevant information, if they are encouraged and motivated to protect their long-term health and if there are no barriers to making those choices. This book sets out the essential information people need, as well as illustrating the benefit of healthy choices and describing how some of the barriers might be overcome. It is particularly appropriate that the book was produced by combining the scientific expertise of the Coronary Prevention Group with the campaigning spirit of Consumers' Association, for if we are to defeat heart disease we need both knowledge and the will to promote it to as wide an audience as possible.

I can commend this book to all those seeking a healthier life for themselves, their families and their communities.

Professor Philip James MA, MD, D.Sc., FRCP, FRCP(E), FRSE, Chairman of the Coronary Prevention Group

ACKNOWLEDGEMENTS

MANY people helped to prepare this book. They found facts (and checked them), read drafts, made helpful comments and, most important, were enthusiastic. It's impossible to name them all but I would like to thank them all – you know who you are!

Only one event marred what had been a very enjoyable experience. Someone very dear to me died of a heart attack just before this book was finished. He was 47 and a great teacher who still had so much to contribute to the world. I shall miss him.

It is this kind of everyday tragedy which brought Consumers' Association and the Coronary Prevention Group together to produce *Preventing Heart Disease*.

Jeanette Longfield

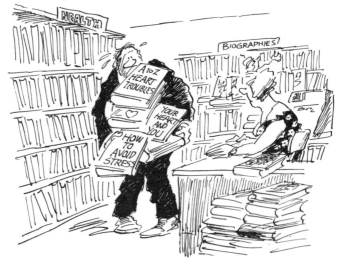

INTRODUCTION

To some extent there will always be a need for a new book about heart disease, if only to bring people up to date with the never-ending stream of new information. Heart disease, like any other human disorder, is complex and difficult to understand. After more than 40 years of scientific investigations, still too little is known about it, so the research continues. This book will provide an overview of the latest research results, together with advice about what people can do to minimise the risk of developing coronary heart disease and advice for people who already have the disease.

A critical look at the great mass of scientific data, both old and new, together with an outline of the way in which information is collected and interpreted, answers questions such as, why do scientists never seem to agree? How can someone who smoked 40 cigarettes a day, never exercised and ate the fattiest foods have lived to be 90? And is there anything you can do nowadays which *isn't* bad for your heart?

This book will also look at what can be done as a society. Choosing a healthy diet is not just a matter of knowing which foods to buy. Your choice may be affected by a wide range of factors, such as the price of different types of products, what you know about the nutritional content of the product from the label and in advertising, how near you are to food shops and what the various members of your household like eating.

Many of these factors are beyond your control. Decisions taken by Government and industry at local, national and international level influence, to some extent, the kinds of food you buy. Public policies across a broad spectrum – not just about food but on matters as diverse as taxation and transport –

may affect your choice. This book also examines the role of these decision-makers in encouraging people to choose a healthier lifestyle.

About the authors

Consumers' Association and the Coronary Prevention Group are perhaps the ideal partners for collaborating on such a book. Consumers' Association is known not only for providing consumers with the independent information they need, but also for making sure that the Government provides the legal framework which will protect consumers from unsafe or shoddy goods, poor services and the like.

But Consumers' Association has to deal with *all* goods and services which interest its members. The Coronary Prevention Group, on the other hand, is devoted solely to the prevention of coronary heart disease. Like Consumers' Association, the Coronary Prevention Group provides independent information and also talks to the policy-makers whose decisions can critically affect what you, the consumer, are able to do. Together, we aim to offer you the best possible chance of preventing heart disease.

Science and heart disease

It is often thought that science is all about 'hard facts' and 'truth', but sometimes it appears that scientists make several different, and even contradictory, statements, causing people to suspect that perhaps all of them are wrong. What follows is a guide to the pros and cons of different types of scientific evidence. One way of looking at science is to see it as detective work – a suspicion is checked out and, if it seems fairly convincing, the scientist or researcher will try to 'prove it'. To take a ridiculous example, a doctor or researcher might notice that most heart disease patients seem to wear black shoes. He or she begins to wonder if there is a connection between black shoes and heart disease. How can this be 'proved'?

Looking at populations

One powerful method of establishing a connection is to look at and compare groups of people – a process called epidemiology. The scientists in our example above may undertake a case-control study: that is, looking at a group of people who have heart disease ('cases') and comparing them to a group of people who don't ('controls') to see whether the cases are more likely to wear black shoes than the controls.

The problem with this type of study is that it is very difficult to choose cases and controls in a way which will not bias the results of the study. It is also more difficult than you might think to diagnose a case of heart disease. The various tests for the most common type of heart disease will be looked at in chapter three of this book, but the relevant question is not so much 'Do I have it or not?' as 'How *much* heart disease do I have.'

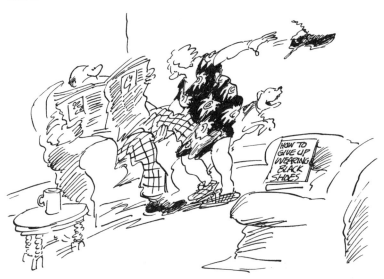

In choosing a control group, researchers have to choose people who are a representative sample of the same group of the population as the cases. This means they should be similar to the cases in almost all respects – age, sex, level of income, educational achievement and so on – so that when the two groups are compared it is possible to spot the key differences which might be linked to heart disease. The two groups must not be exactly the same. The epidemiologist Geoffrey Rose of the London School of Hygiene and Tropical Medicine pointed out that if everyone in the world had smoked it would have been impossible to spot the link between smoking and disease. Since non-smokers can act as controls, an enormous number of studies have been able to show the links between smoking and a whole range of diseases.

Cases and controls should not be completely different either because this would make comparisons impossible. It is also best to exclude from the groups any known differences, called confounding variables, which might affect the disease being studied. For example, exercise can reduce the risk of heart disease, so the results of a case-control study on heart disease would not be useful if, unknown to the research group, the control group were all marathon runners. Despite all these drawbacks, case-control studies can provide useful evidence to back up a hunch. They provide the kind of circumstantial evidence that might help researchers to focus their ideas on a particular suspect cause.

Another way to back up the hunch is to do a cross-sectional study. One of the earliest examples of this type of study in the field of heart disease, and still one of the most famous, was done in the early 1950s by Professor Ancel Keys, from Minneapolis in the United States. The study looking at 16 groups of men aged 40 to 59 in seven countries: Finland, Greece, Italy, Japan, the Netherlands, the United States and Yugoslavia. Over 12,000 men were studied to see whether they showed signs of coronary heart disease, and to see what factors might be linked to the presence (or absence) of the disease. The results showed that the amount of cholesterol in the blood is a vital factor in heart disease. Keys' Seven Countries Study also showed that blood cholesterol levels seemed to be strongly linked to the amount of saturated fat in the diet.

The results from Ancel Keys' research show a broad trend: the higher the percentage of calories from saturated fat, the higher the blood cholesterol levels. This type of study cannot, however, explain some of the discrepancies that came to light.

For example, why did the group of Yugoslavian men have roughly the same amount of saturated fat in their diet as the men in Crete, but a much lower blood cholesterol level?

With a clearer idea of what they are looking for, scientists might decide to do a prospective study (also sometimes known as a cohort, or longitudinal study). In this type of population study two or more groups of people with different exposure to the suspect factor are studied over a long period of time. The British Regional Heart Study, for example, is looking at almost 8,000 men aged 40 to 59 in 24 towns all over Britain and is collecting information on factors such as smoking, blood pressure and blood cholesterol. With sophisticated statistical techniques and computer technology, it is possible to isolate each factor and calculate how closely it is associated with heart disease.

So far, we have looked at surveys which describe what is happening in different groups of the population – by comparing people with heart disease against people without heart disease (case-control studies), or by looking at very large samples of people (cross-sectional studies), or by studying cohorts of people over a long period of time (prospective studies). These methods provide circumstantial evidence to support the basic hunch that the suspect factor might cause heart disease. Even if the links are very strong, it cannot be proved that any of the factors actually *causes* heart disease. The studies can only show links and associations.

Going back to the black shoe example, if the factor of black shoes really is a cause of heart disease then you would expect that the incidence of heart disease would increase with the numbers of people wearing black shoes, and if people stopped wearing them, or wore them less often, then the incidence of heart disease would be less frequent. In the fourth type of population study, researchers actually intervene to see if reducing the suspect factor will reduce the incidence of heart disease, hence the term intervention studies. Sometimes the intervention is accidental. During the Second World War many countries were forced to introduce rationing on items such as meat and butter – foods which are high in saturated fat. Looking back at medical records for that time, there was a sharp drop in deaths from heart disease. In the United States, where there was no rationing at that time, heart disease rates continued to climb.

This still falls short of a proven cause of heart disease, but scientists began to design studies which introduced changes deliberately. One example of this approach was the MRFIT (or Multiple Risk Factor Intervention Trial) study in the United States, which involved the study of almost 13,000 men aged 35 to 57. They were chosen because, being smokers with higher than average blood pressure and blood cholesterol levels, they were at a higher than average risk of developing heart disease. About half the men were given 'ordinary' care by their doctors and the other half were given special attention to try and reduce their risk.

After seven years of the MRFIT study, the special care group were smoking less and had lower blood pressure and cholesterol levels than the ordinary group. Slightly fewer of them died from heart disease. The problem for the researchers was that the ordinary group had changed their behaviour more than expected. They, too, were smoking less, and taking care with their diet and so on. Their rates of coronary heart disease were lower then predicted; in fact the rates were almost the same as those of the control groups. The major drawback with all intervention studies, therefore, is that in real life it is difficult to control the control group.

In the laboratory

Under laboratory conditions it is possible to keep almost everything under control. By varying a single element at a time it is possible to observe exactly what influence that element has on the result. It is at this level, where the elusive proof of whether the suspect factor causes heart disease, comes closest. These studies also come in different forms, with their own strengths and weaknesses. For example, epidemiological studies have shown a strong link between eating too much saturated fat and incidence of heart disease. Researchers can look at the effect of saturated fat on the human body as a whole, or on the heart in particular, or on detailed parts of the heart, or on the cells inside those parts or even on the molecules inside the cells. Some of this research can be done with human volunteers, for example people who have moderate or severe coronary heart disease; some research must be done post mortem, or on various kinds of animals; other types can be performed on cells grown in a laboratory. But even these very detailed scientific experiments can fail to provide the elusive proof. Arguments still rage in the scientific community about the relevance of animal experiments for humans. Looking at organs, or tissues, or cells in isolation might not explain exactly how they work in a living human being in a complex world.

All of the drawbacks to scientific methods outlined so far apply to studies which have been designed and carried out thoroughly, and to the highest standards – they are 'good science'. Yet scientists are only human, so some studies are based on sounder research methods than others. For example, our researchers interested in the black shoe theory may only have looked at a couple of dozen heart disease patients – nowhere near enough people for any conclusions to be drawn about the whole population. Or the research definitions may not have been drawn carefully enough, leading the scientists to look at very dark brown shoes as well as black ones.

These are just some of the reasons why scientists seem never to agree. They may be looking at different questions or using different methods. Even if they obtain similar results they may choose to interpret them differently, or draw very firm conclusions from quite weak results. Add to all this the complication of media coverage of science. It is too easy to blame television and newspapers for being sensational and unbalanced. Journalists seek out new angles, arguments and evidence; when researchers publish the results of their latest survey or experiment, a journalist will want to focus in his or her report on what is different.

In a short news story or a brief column, there probably will not be space for explaining all the background, the pros and cons, or whether it is 'good' or 'bad' science. Many journalists have no scientific background and, given the fact that they are in competition with other reporters and have tight deadlines to meet, they are unlikely to have time to check the facts with experts. Stories sometimes get into the news in advance of publication of the full facts, or a journalist might pick up an off-the-cuff comment from a researcher. So the difference between studies can end up being exaggerated out of all proportion.

The diversity of science and scientists can be seen as a weakness because it cannot provide absolute proof, but it is also a strength. Each scientist or group of researchers may have their own pet theory which they believe provides the best explanation for what causes heart disease. But every result is closely scrutinised by other scientists. If something new or unexpected is revealed by research, it sparks off more studies designed to probe, until it is either dismissed as a freak result or confirmed as another possible lead to follow.

After many years of research into heart disease the experts *do* agree so, as heart disease is examined in this book, each part will answer the same key questions that scientists would ask: first, how strong is the link? Is the circumstantial evidence strong and consistent across all types of study? Weak or inconsistent links, or results which are too new to be checked against others, will be treated with caution. Second, is the link a likely cause? Is there a plausible explanation in biology, chemistry or physics that the link may be a cause? If not, it might be just a coincidence. To go back to our ridiculous example, surveys might show a link between people wearing black shoes and heart disease, but it is so unlikely that black shoes cause heart disease that this link is most probably mere chance.

Deciding what to do

How can you translate general scientific statements about heart disease and its suspected risk factors into sensible advice about what you as an individual should do? The problem is that every individual has his or her own unique combination of heart disease risks, made up of inherited factors and a whole range of other influences. It is not yet clear why your friend's cousin's grandmother Doris smoked 40 cigarettes a day, had fried bacon and eggs every morning for breakfast and lived to the age of 93. Nor do we know exactly why your aunt's friend's neighbour Fred, for example, who never smoked in his life, was a vegetarian and who cycled to work every day, died of a heart attack at 52. More and more of the secrets of heart disease are being unlocked by science but what we *do* know already is that if you took 100 'Doris-type' people and 100 'Fred-type' people, more members of the 'Doris' group would not see their 90s than those of the 'Fred group'. Each person will balance the risks and benefits of doing nothing, or doing something, about heart disease. The third and final key question for each section of the book: after 'how strong is the link?' and 'is it a likely cause?' comes 'what are the risks and benefits?' Everything we do has risks and benefits – life itself is a risky business but it is possible to make reasonable calculations about risks and benefits to see which is the best possible option. The changes in diet and lifestyle made in order to reduce the risk of coronary heart disease may help to prevent other diseases and conditions, such as some types of cancer, diabetes and obesity, and also improve your general health.

Government, industry, the media, and the professions can all change the balance of risks and benefits in a way which might influence what you choose to do. Take smoking, for example. You might well have been considering giving up. Then Budget Day comes round and there's a sizeable increase in tobacco taxes. It proves to be just the helping hand you needed to stop smoking for good. There is good evidence that higher taxation stops people smoking on quite a large scale, so that for every 10 per cent increase in price there is a 5 per cent fall in cigarette consumption. Similarly if there is no tax increase, or just a small one, the incentive to give up smoking is lost.

This is just one example of how the actions of others can affect what you do. In fact, there is a wide range of policy choices facing Government, industry and the professions (see chapter ten). These policies, together with consumer action, hold the potential to effect a substantial decline in the UK's appallingly high rates of death and disability from coronary heart disease.

CHAPTER 1

YOUR HEART AND HOW IT WORKS

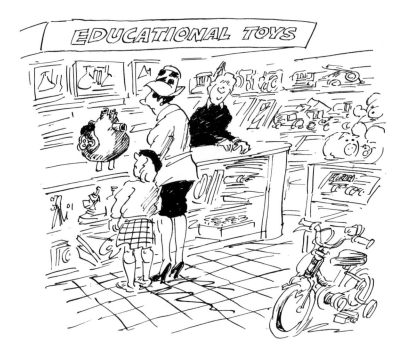

The heart is a pump with four hollow chambers. Two chambers mainly collect the blood – the left atrium (marked as 1 on the diagram) and the right atrium (marked as 3 on the diagram). 'Atrium' is Latin for hall. The other two chambers are for pumping the blood – the left ventricle (number 2) and the right ventricle (number 4).

When a person breathes in oxygen flows into the lungs, where it is absorbed by the blood which becomes bright red. The red, oxygen-rich blood leaves the lungs and flows through the pulmonary veins ('pulmo' means lung in Latin) into the heart.

Your Heart and How it Works

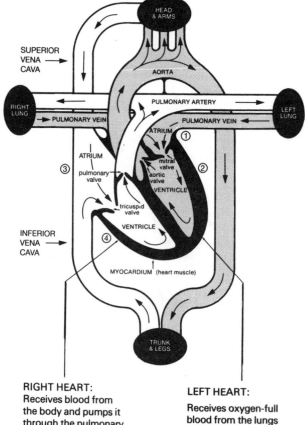

RIGHT HEART:
Receives blood from the body and pumps it through the pulmonary artery to the lungs where it picks up fresh oxygen and gives off carbon dioxide.

LEFT HEART:
Receives oxygen-full blood from the lungs and pumps it through the aorta to the body.

From the left atrium the blood goes through the first of four valves. All the valves in the heart are there to make sure that the blood keeps flowing in a forward direction. This first valve is called the mitral valve because, with its two flaps, early scientists thought it looked rather like a bishop's mitre.

The blood flows down the left atrium through the mitral valve into the left ventricle (number 2). The blood is pumped out of the left ventricle through the second valve – the aortic valve – into the aorta. The aorta is the main artery in the body and all the other arteries branch off from this one, taking the blood with oxygen and nutrients to all the parts of the body.

Here the blood gives up its oxygen and other nutrients and collects waste products and carbon dioxide. The blood loses its red colour and turns bluish. This much darker-coloured blood flows into the veins and begins its journey back to the heart.

The veins from the head and arms eventually join up to form the superior vena cava. In Latin 'vena' is vein, 'cava' is hollow and superior means that it is higher up. The veins from the legs and the body become the inferior vena cava – the hollow vein lower down. The bluish blood from these two large veins then flows into the right atrium (number 3) and down through the third heart valve – the tricuspid valve ('tri' comes from the Latin for three), so called because it has three flaps or 'cusps'.

Having flowed through the tricuspid valve, the blood arrives in the right ventricle (number 4). From here, the blood carrying the carbon dioxide is pumped out through the last valve, the pulmonary valve, into the pulmonary artery which divides in two to go back to the lungs. When the person breathes out carbon dioxide is released from the lungs into the air.

Heart beats

When the body is resting the heart beats 60 to 70 times a minute, which means that the procedure described above takes less than one second. When exercising, the healthy heart can comfortably manage 160 to 180 beats every minute, so the process can happen two or three times every second.

The number of beats is controlled automatically by the sinus node, the heart's own pacemaker. This pacemaker is a group of cells in the top right-hand side of the heart (i.e. the right atrium) which can send electrical signals to other parts of the heart. One pulse or beat from the pacemaker sets off the following sequence in the heart.

As the left atrium and the right atrium (the atria) contract at the same time, they open their respective valves and let the blood flow down into the left and right ventricles before the valves close again. A mere fraction of a second later, that same electrical pulse or beat makes the muscle walls of the ventricles contract and push the blood out to the body and lungs. The delay is caused by the electrical pulse going through a kind of junction box which separates the atria from the ventricles. It is called the atrioventricular or AV node. This electrical pulse from the pacemaker which makes the atria and ventricles of the heart contract in rapid sequence to push the blood round the system is called systole.

After systole there is a short pause before the next pulse or heart beat. This pause is called diastole (see page 23).

The pacemaker speeds up or slows down in response to signals from the body and yet it still keeps a regular rhythm. Reflexes, hormones and other body chemicals can affect the pacemaker and tell it, for example, to slow down when the body is asleep or to speed up when running to catch the train. So this is how the heart works – the most efficient pump in the world – beating some 100,000 times a day, every day, for the whole of our lives.

Blood pressure

To be more precise we should really say that the heart is *two* pumps working side by side, separated by the atrial septum (Latin for wall) and the ventricular septum.

The blood held in the left and right atria is only being pumped as far as the ventricles below so the atria don't need very strong pumping muscles. The left ventricle has to push the blood through the main artery to the whole of the body so this chamber has thick muscular walls and is a very strong pump.

The blood in the arteries is pushed very hard – in other words, it is under pressure. If there was no pressure in the arteries, the blood would never reach all the parts of the body.

The arteries need to be strong enough to withstand the pressure but also stretchy enough to cope with the fact that the pressure comes in pulses, in time with the heart beat. So the arteries are not just hollow tubes, they have four layers to give strength and flexibility: a fibrous outer coating, a muscular wall, an elastic layer and a smooth, delicate inner lining. These tough and stretchy arteries divide into smaller and smaller branches that are called arterioles.

Each time the heart beats and the blood surges through, the arteries and arterioles expand a little. This is the blood pressure at its highest point and, since it coincides with the systole sequence of the heart (i.e. when it beats), it is called systolic pressure. During diastole, when the heart chambers and the arteries are relaxing, blood pressure is at its lowest point and is called diastolic pressure.

In the same way as the heart can speed up or slow down according to the demands of the day, the blood pressure in the arteries and arterioles can also vary. The level of pressure is determined by two main factors: the amount of blood being pumped with each heart beat and how much resistance there is in the arterioles. In other words, if the arterioles don't expand enough to let the blood through, the heart has to work harder to push the blood round the system. Blood pressure is higher, for example, when you are excited (your heart is pumping faster and pumping more blood with each beat and your arterioles are 'tight') and lower when you are resting, for example, watching a boring TV programme (your heart is at its resting rate and the arterioles are relaxed). These temporary ups and downs in the level of blood pressure in the arteries and arterioles are quite normal and a healthy body can cope with these fluctuations easily.

Blood pressure is permanently much lower when the blood moves onto the next stage of its journey round the body.

From the tiny arteries or arterioles, blood flows into even finer tubes called capillaries. These hair-like capillaries are only one layer thick and, because the blood in the arteries is at the end of its journey, there is a drop in blood pressure. Oxygen and nutrients simply seep out through the walls of the capillaries into the body's tissues.

The capillaries are also the points from which the blood starts its circuit back to the heart. Waste products and carbon dioxide drain from the tissues into adjoining capillaries, giving the blood a bluish tinge. The capillaries drain first into small veins, then into larger veins and finally into the two largest veins, the superior vena cava and the inferior vena cava, before entering the right side of the heart.

Because the system of veins is under much lower pressure than the arteries the veins are thinner and less elastic and have only three layers to the arteries' four. The right side of the heart needs a much less powerful pump than the left side as a circuit round the lungs is a good deal less taxing for the right ventricle than pumping blood round the whole body. After the blood flows into the top right-hand chamber of the heart – the atrium – it flows through the tricuspid valve into the right ventricle and is pumped through the pulmonary valve to the lungs, where the carbon dioxide can be breathed out.

Back to the heart of the matter

An average of five litres (about 11 pints) of blood constantly circulates through the heart and body. The heart can pump the entire five litres all the way round in a minute or less – the equivalent of around 7,000 litres (roughly 1,540 gallons) in a day. It is not surprising, then, that the heart's own muscles and tissues need a good supply of blood, with the oxygen and nutrients it carries, to keep them in good condition. This blood supply does not come from the thousands of litres flowing through the heart each day: the heart has its own supply.

The heart's arteries branch off from the main artery – the aorta – and lie on the surface of the heart. There are two arteries on the heart muscle or myocardium: one for each side of the heart. But, since the left side of the heart has the largest pumping muscle, the left artery divides into two almost immediately, with one branch going round the back of the heart, so they are normally referred to as the three main arteries. These three arteries divide into smaller and smaller branches which penetrate deep into the heart muscle, so that the heart gets a rich supply of blood. When they were first discovered scientists thought the arteries circled the heart rather like a crown. The Latin for crown is 'corona', hence the term coronary arteries.

CHAPTER 2

WHAT CAN GO WRONG?

DESPITE of its complex structure, and the extraordinary amount of work it has to do over a lifetime, the heart rarely goes wrong. Most people get many thousands of hours of excellent service from their 'wonder pump'. Unfortunately, too many people do not.

Heart disease comes in many different forms. The most common type of heart disease in Britain, and in other Western countries, is coronary heart disease. In the Third World rheumatic heart disease is a major problem. There are also several other cardiac disorders, not related to coronary heart disease or rheumatic heart disease, which we shall also describe in lesser detail.

For some types of heart disease the reasons why the heart stops working properly remain a mystery. Even though the causes of these heart diseases have not yet been discovered, there are some remarkable and effective treatments. Scientists and researchers have some very strong clues, however, about the causes of coronary heart disease, clues which allow us much greater potential for preventing it.

Coronary heart disease

Coronary heart disease is the most common type of heart disease in Britain. In 1989, 92,480 men and 76,421 women died from coronary heart disease, an average of 460 people every day. By the time you finish reading this page another person could well have been added to the toll. The tragedy of coronary heart disease is that it often affects people before they ever get to enjoy their retirement: this type of heart disease accounts for one in three of all deaths in men before the age of 65 and one in seven of all deaths in women under 65. It can also cause a great deal of pain and distress.

It may seem as though coronary heart disease does indeed 'strike like a bolt out of the blue', but it does not. It takes many years for coronary heart disease to develop and though we still do not have all the pieces of the coronary heart disease 'puzzle', we have enough to be able to see the basic picture.

Atherosclerosis

Transportation of oxygen to all parts of the body by the blood is only one function of this vital fluid. It also carries nutrients to the tissues in the body. Some of these nutrients come from the food we eat (see chapter six) and some are made by the body itself. The nutrients that are relevant to coronary heart disease are fats, also known as lipids.

Because blood is mostly water, and fat and water don't mix, the body has to bind the fat to something else so that it can be carried by the blood. The different types of fat, or lipids, are bound together with protein to form particles called lipoproteins. There are different types of lipoproteins and the 'baddies', in terms of coronary heart disease, are low density lipoproteins, or LDLs. Their job is to take blood lipids, particularly cholesterol, to the body's cells. Cholesterol is taken away from the cells by high density lipoproteins, or HDLs, and these HDLs are often referred to as 'good' cholesterol.

Cholesterol is a soft, waxy material that is an essential part of all the cells in the body. It is used, for example, to make hormones and substances in the nervous system. The problem with cholesterol is that if the liver cannot dispose of it effectively, it starts to build up in the blood and, when carried by the LDLs, it sometimes 'sticks' to the inside surface of the arteries.

As cholesterol circulates in the body, the previously smooth lining of the arteries starts to develop fatty streaks of cholesterol. This process can start very early in life and has been found in the arteries of children who died in accidents. Young American soldiers who died in the Korean war in the 1950s were found to have quite well advanced fatty streaks. The same streaks were found in the arteries of Americans killed in Vietnam in the 1960s. Although these fatty streaks don't necessarily develop, over the years they may become bigger and thicker and eventually develop into patches or plaques in the arteries. Other substances such as calcium may stick to them, so that the plaques can become hard and brittle.

Sometimes the plaques crack, and bleed inside the artery. Just as when you cut your finger, the blood forms clots to stop the bleeding and help the cut heal, so clots can form inside the artery to heal the plaques. Unfortunately, this can make the plaques even bigger, taking up more room inside the artery and leaving less room for the blood to flow through. The process by which plaques form and develop is called atherosclerosis. The Greek word 'athare', meaning porridge, is a fitting description of the pale, lumpy substance which builds up. The Greek word 'skleros', meaning hardening, completes the vivid picture of dried porridge furring up the arteries: arteriosclerosis or hardening of the arteries.

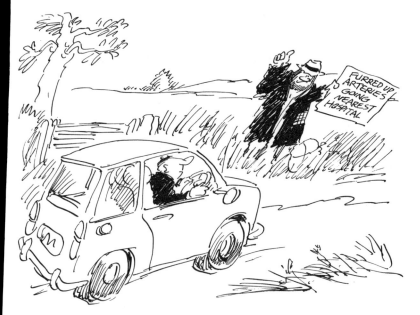

In chapter one the importance of a good supply of oxygen-rich blood for the heart was established. So if the heart's own arteries, the coronary arteries, begin to suffer from atherosclerosis the heart starts to get less blood than it needs to work properly. Atherosclerosis in the coronary arteries has a number of other names including coronary artery disease and ischaemic heart disease (from the Greek 'iskheim', meaning to hold back and 'haima' meaning blood). So coronary artery disease describes the process of atherosclerosis and coronary heart disease describes the effects on the sufferer. It is possible, though not very common, to have quite bad coronary artery disease and not feel any ill effects at all. This is known as silent ischaemia. More commonly, you will begin to feel ill effects if there is an increase in the work the heart has to do, for example, if you do something strenuous. The heart will beat faster and will need more oxygen to do the extra work but because the coronary arteries are furred up with atherosclerosis the blood is unable to squeeze through fast enough.

Angina

The pain produced when the heart muscle cannot get enough oxygen is known as angina, or angina pectoris (combining the Greek word for strangling, 'agkheim', with the Latin word for chest, 'pectus'). Sometimes the pain can be just a twinge, but it can be much worse. One book on heart disease has described it as 'like having an elephant sitting on your chest'! The main feature of ordinary or stable angina is that, once the strenuous event that brought on the attack has finished, the pain goes away after a few minutes. No permanent damage is done to the heart because oxygen-rich blood can still get to all the parts of the heart, even if it is only trickling through instead of flowing as freely as it should.

There is a small group of people who suffer from the symptoms of heart disease – angina, for example – but who, after medical investigation, turn out to have no atherosclerosis in their coronary arteries. The cause of their pain is exactly the same – the heart muscle isn't getting enough oxygen – but it is not because the arteries are permanently narrowed by atherosclerosis but because sections of their arteries become temporarily narrowed. It is not known what triggers this temporary narrowing or coronary artery spasm.

Heart attack

Another possible problem for someone with coronary artery disease is that one or more of the arteries becomes so narrow that, the next time a plaque bursts and a clot forms to heal it, the clot actually blocks off the artery completely. This is often called a coronary thrombosis. It can cause a myocardial infarct or infarction (heart attack). As the blood can no longer flow through the artery, the heart muscle (or myocardium) beyond it begins to die, or infarct. This is the most common form of heart attack. The pain of a heart attack does not go away after a few moments' rest and permanent damage is done to the heart muscle. The extent of the damage and the intensity of the pain depend on where the blockage forms. If it is quite near the bottom of the heart, in one of the smaller arteries, then only a small section of heart muscle will be damaged. In time the heart can even grow new arteries, albeit small ones, to bypass the blocked artery. These arteries are called collaterals. If the blockage was near the origin of one of the three main coronary arteries, then the resultant damage could be very serious indeed. A terrible crushing pain can spread from the chest to the neck and arms. For some people, it is the last thing they ever feel.

Complications after a heart attack

Sudden death is often caused, not by the heart attack itself, but by a complication that arises from it. When part of the heart muscle dies, particularly if that part is large, the heart's natural rhythm can be disturbed. The ventricles, instead of beating regularly, can start to quiver or flutter. This is called ventricular fibrillation and it can be fatal, since it means that no blood is being pumped round the body and to any vital organs such as the brain and the heart itself.

It is possible literally to shock the heart so that it stops fluttering and starts to beat rhythmically again. The machines that can do this are called defibrillators, but to be successful the machine has to reach the person suffering the attack very quickly indeed. All hospitals have defibrillators and all frontline ambulances will soon be equipped with them. GPs' surgeries sometimes have defibrillators too, but sadly, for many people, it is too late for the machine to be used.

Why is it that atherosclerosis affects the coronary arteries? No one is quite sure, but it seems likely that the furring up process may start (and be aggravated) where the smooth and thin inner lining of the arteries becomes damaged. Since the heart muscle is the only one in the body in constant motion, and the arteries on its surface are forever being squeezed and released by the heart's contractions, they might be more prone to this kind of minor damage. Because they are so small, the coronary arteries may be more vulnerable to being furred up by atheroma or blocked by clots. After all, the heart is only about the size of a clenched fist, so even its main arteries are no wider than a small drinking straw. Other factors such as smoking and high blood pressure can also damage the arteries (see chapter three).

But all the arteries in the body can be affected by the narrowing and clotting process of atherosclerosis. Sometimes the clots which form can break off and be swept into the bloodstream, only to lodge in a narrower artery and cause a blockage there. These moving clots are called embolisms. If any of these problems occur in or near the arteries of the brain a stroke occurs and, like heart attacks, these can be fatal.

Peripheral arterial disease

As angina occurs when the heart cannot get enough oxygen, the same thing can happen in the legs if the arteries are deprived of oxygen. This problem is called peripheral arterial disease. When walking, for example, the leg muscles need more oxygen to do the extra work, but because the leg arteries are furred up or blocked, the oxygen-rich blood cannot reach the muscles and a cramp-like pain develops. As with angina, this pain fades after a few moments' rest, but it can return later in the walk. This occasional pain in the legs is known as intermittent claudication, after the Emperor Claudius, who had a limp. This type of pain in the legs should *not* be regarded as a sign that you ought to stop walking. In fact, the more you walk the more likely it is that your muscles will develop collaterals, or new arteries, to get around the blockage, just as they can in the heart muscle. In some cases, peripheral arterial disease can become more serious than this, leading to death of the leg muscles, gangrene and even necessitating amputation.

Congenital heart disease

Congenital heart disease affects very few people – only eight babies in every 1,000 born – and scientists have very little idea about what causes it. Congenital heart disease is actually an umbrella term for a number of different heart problems which can result in death and disability. Around 5,000 babies are born with congenital heart disease each year and some 1,000 of these will die soon after they are born. The heart defects of about 2,000 babies are not serious and no treatment at all is necessary. Even for the remaining 2,000 babies, most problems can be successfully treated, or at least improved, with modern drugs and surgical techniques, so the outlook for them is very good.

One of the most common forms of congenital heart disease is known as a 'hole in the heart'. The baby is born with a hole in the wall, or septum, dividing the left and right side of the heart. This causes the red, oxygen-rich blood to mix with the bluish blood carrying the carbon dioxide, spoiling the one-way flow round the body and reducing the level of oxygen in the arterial blood. The hole can often heal up by itself. If it does not, then it can be closed successfully by surgery.

Another common problem is patent ductus arteriosus. Before birth, the baby 'breathes' from its mother's lungs, via the placenta, so the baby's pulmonary arteries, which would normally take blood (and oxygen) to its own lungs, have a channel or duct which bypasses the lungs. This duct usually closes up as soon as the baby takes its first breath. When it does not, drugs or surgery can put the fault right.

It is particularly important with congenital heart disease to be scrupulous with childhood infections, in order to help avoid future complications. Cuts which turn septic, boils or infected teeth and gums, can all allow bacteria that may attack the affected part of the heart to enter the bloodstream. Always tell the dentist about the child's heart problem even if it has completely cleared up.

Rubella

There are various other congenital defects that can occur singly, or, in more serious cases, together. Several viruses and a range of other factors, such as Down's Syndrome and the drugs thalidomide and lithium, have been associated with birth defects in general and congenital heart disease in particular. German measles, or rubella, is also a known cause of congenital heart disease. If the mother comes into contact with German measles during the first three months of pregnancy there is a strong likelihood of problems developing in the baby. The message is clear: if you are planning to become pregnant, ask your doctor to make absolutely sure that you have a resistance to this infection. If you are not immune, make sure you are inoculated before you become pregnant. If you are pregnant and come into contact with someone with rubella, consult your doctor at once.

Diseases of the heart valves

If something goes wrong with the four heart valves, the heart's ability to pump blood effectively round the body can be seriously reduced. Valve diseases may be due to congenital abnormalities, rheumatic fever (see opposite) or bacterial infection. Fortunately, heart valve problems can be put right fairly simply and they rarely cause difficulties for people in Britain. If something does go wrong, it is usually with the valves on the left side of the heart (the mitral valve and the aortic valve), since they have the most work to do. The problems come in two main forms: stenosis (from the Greek 'stenos', meaning to narrow) where the valve literally becomes too narrow and stiff and cannot open properly to let the blood flow through; and incompetence, where the valve becomes incapable of doing its job, letting blood leak backwards instead of going forwards in just one direction. A better term for describing this is regurgitation. Occasionally valves can be both leaky and narrow, neither opening nor closing properly.

If these problems are allowed to develop untreated, heart failure can result (see page 37). Usually, the problem can be improved with drugs or corrected by surgery to replace or repair the problem valve. Around 5,000 valves are replaced every year in the UK and the replacements can be made either from animal tissue or from artificial materials such as plastic or metal.

Rheumatic heart disease

The good news is that in Britain at least, we have already prevented many future problems from valve disease. The medical world has long been aware that the cause of most valve problems is rheumatic fever. Thirty or more years ago it was still quite common in the UK and many people who have valve disease today suffered from rheumatic fever when they were children. The fever begins as a bacterial infection (streptococcus) which gives the sufferer a sore throat and a nasty fever for two or three weeks. A poisonous by-product of the bacteria can attack the heart valves, leaving them scarred and weakened so that later in life the valves are liable to cause the kind of problems described above. The conditions in which bacteria thrive – gross overcrowding in poor housing conditions, poor hygiene and low resistance to infection due to poor nutrition – are no longer common in this country. Thanks to the National Health Service it has also become much easier to get prompt medical treatment for any infection that does take hold. In years to come we can look forward to a sharp drop in the number of people with diseases of the heart valve.

Unfortunately there will still be a few cases of valve disease. Sometimes, for reasons we simply do not understand, the heart valves seem to wear out in old age, or a faulty valve can be one of the forms of congenital heart disease. But for everyone who has valve problems, whatever the cause, it is important to have regular check-ups – even though you feel fine – to make sure that any deterioration can be caught and corrected in time.

It is also important to take good care of your teeth and gums, for the same reason that children with congenital heart disease should do so: mouth infections can let bacteria into the bloodstream, which then attack the weakened valve. Make sure you tell your dentist about any valve problems and, if dental surgery is necessary, antibiotics should prevent any mishaps.

Palpitations or abnormal heart rhythms

Palpitations in the heart can feel very frightening. It is comforting to know that they are rarely serious and can usually be treated very successfully. The problem is a fault in the heart's electrical system – the pacemaker – so that instead of beating steadily the heart beats get out of rhythm (arrhythmia).

Sometimes the heart begins to beat far too slowly, a condition called bradycardia (from the Greek word for slow, 'bradus'). Occasionally heart block develops, in which the pulses from the pacemaker don't pass through the junction box to reach the ventricles. Because the ventricles, particularly the left one, are so important, the heart has a back-up system which keeps the ventricles pumping automatically and without the electrical pulse from the pacemaker. Unfortunately the pumping action is very slow (only 30 beats per minute). This is sometimes enough to keep you alive, but as it is not enough for you to be able to *do* anything, treatment is necessary. This is usually in the form of an artificial pacemaker and is very successful. Technology has advanced so rapidly that there are now hundreds of models to choose from and thousands of pacemakers are fitted every year.

Another rhythm problem is that the heart begins to beat far too fast. This is called tachycardia ('takhus' means swift in Greek). This is not the same as the fibrillation that can happen during a heart attack, which is utterly unco-ordinated and very dangerous. During an attack of tachycardia the heart's rhythm is maintained, but it simply beats more quickly than is necessary. This problem can often be controlled with drugs.

Finally, there are times when the heart seems to miss a beat and, because the beat seems to be out of place, they are called ectopic beats, after the Greek word for 'displaced', 'ektopos'. Most people have probably had this sensation from time to time and it is not thought to be serious. Some people find that ectopic beats are brought on by drinking strong tea, coffee or alcohol, in which case it is probably best to avoid these drinks. Usually, though, there is no apparent reason for these odd beats.

Some rhythm disorders can be brought on by a heart attack or follow heart surgery. Other rhythm problems can be caused by rheumatic heart disease (see page 35) or an over-active thyroid gland.

Heart failure

Coronary heart disease can lead to heart failure. If a very large section of heart muscle dies after a heart attack, or if the heart has insufficient time to recover after several attacks, the heart muscle may become too weak to pump properly. Damage to the left side is the most serious and, as the pumping action weakens and the blood begins to collect in the chamber instead of flowing out to the body, the blood begins to back up along the pulmonary veins that feed the heart from the lungs. Eventually the blood backs up into the lungs themselves, seeping out into the lungs to make them 'water-logged' or congested, and breathing becomes very difficult. Occasionally the right pumping chamber can be affected. When this happens blood cannot drain back properly from the veins into the heart. Blood backs up in the veins and fluid builds up, particularly in the ankles, making them swell. In very serious cases both the left and right sides of the heart fail to pump properly.

The same problem can happen if valve disease is not caught in time. The heart muscles may simply give up the long battle against stiff and/or leaky valves and, depending on which valve or valves are faulty, congested lungs or swollen limbs can develop.

Drugs can sometimes help to relieve the symptoms of heart failure but the most important line of attack is to deal with the underlying cause, where it is known: coronary heart disease, valve disease or a serious alcohol problem.

Cardiomyopathy

Another mystery in heart disease is the condition known as cardiomyopathy, a term which covers a range of other diseases of the heart muscle, for which there is no known cause (although it can sometimes be caused by the heart muscle being poisoned by excessive alcohol). The heart muscle gets bigger and eventually grows so large that it outgrows its own blood supply. The coronary arteries cannot keep up, and the pumping action starts to fail, with all the consequences already described.

CHAPTER 3

WHAT ARE THE RISKS?

IT IS not clear why coronary heart disease affects some individuals more than others, but it has been established that some factors are very closely linked with coronary heart disease. When one or more of these factors is present, the risk of developing coronary heart disease is very much higher, so they are known as risk factors.

Blood cholesterol

How strong is the link?

The link between coronary heart disease and the amount of cholesterol in the blood is perhaps one of the most researched topics in the whole area of coronary heart disease (see page 28). Professor Ancel Keys' study of seven countries (see page 12) began in the 1950s and showed very clearly that the more cholesterol there was in the blood the more likely it was that coronary heart disease would develop. Since then, many more studies have looked at different countries and at different groups of people in the same country over a number of years. Framingham in the USA, Gothenburg in Sweden, Puerto Rico, and London are just a few of the places where some of the inhabitants have been studied in great detail in this way.

Virtually every study confirmed Professor Keys' suggestion that blood cholesterol is an important element in coronary heart disease. Intervention studies designed to test the theory that rates of coronary heart disease fall if blood cholesterol levels fall seem to show that this is indeed the case. The MRFIT study in America (see page 14) persuaded thousands of American men to change their habits to reduce their blood cholesterol levels and the rates of coronary heart disease fell. Although they didn't fall more than was evident the men who *hadn't* received special advice it seemed to be due to the fact that these men changed their habits too. There were similar results from a project in Finland, where, until fairly recently, coronary heart disease rates were the highest in the world. Around 180,000 people living in North Karelia in Finland were studied for ten years and many different methods were used to persuade people to change their habits so that their blood cholesterol levels would fall. The people of North Karelia were compared with other regions of Finland and, sure enough, the North Karelians did better than people in the rest of Finland at reducing their blood cholesterol levels and their death rates from coronary heart disease. Here again, though, the other Finns reduced their blood cholesterol levels and their rates of coronary heart disease also fell.

Taking the Finnish and American research, together with a number of other similar projects, it has been calculated by Dr Peto (see page 183) that for every one per cent drop in blood cholesterol levels there will be a fall in coronary heart disease rates of two or three per cent. No one has yet found a country where blood cholesterol levels are low and coronary heart disease rates are high. Without raised levels of blood cholesterol, it seems that coronary heart disease does not occur: it is a necessary condition for the development of the disease.

But there are other studies which show that raised blood cholesterol is not a sufficient condition for coronary heart disease. In other words, raised blood cholesterol on its own does not always lead to coronary heart disease. For example, there is a nomadic tribe in the north of Kenya which has blood cholesterol levels very similar to those in Western countries. Yet members of the tribe show no signs of coronary heart disease.

Even Keys' Seven Countries Study showed that countries with the same levels of blood cholesterol could have different rates of coronary heart disease. And in the UK, men employed in the white-collar jobs seem to have higher blood cholesterol levels even though they have lower rates of coronary heart disease than blue-collar workers. Clearly there is more to the story of coronary heart disease than blood cholesterol.

Is blood cholesterol a likely cause?

We have already seen in chapter two (on page 28) how cholesterol is carried in the blood – by HDLs which carry cholesterol away from cells to the liver for disposal, and by LDLs which carry cholesterol to the cells. Scientists have shown how, once the lining of the artery is damaged, LDLs can leave some of their cholesterol stuck to the artery wall. This cholesterol builds up into fatty streaks that can grow into lumps of 'hard porridge,' narrowing the artery and making it more difficult for the blood to flow through (atherosclerosis). Logically, the more cholesterol there is in the blood, particularly when it is carried by the LDLs, the more likely it is that some of the cholesterol will become stuck to the artery walls.

High blood pressure
How strong is the link?

If coronary heart disease cannot be explained in terms of blood cholesterol alone, other risk factors must be involved. The Framingham Heart Study is one of many surveys which showed that the higher the level of blood pressure, the higher the rates of coronary heart disease. In 1948 when the study began, Framingham was a small town on the east coast of America and 5,000 men and women aged between 39 and 50 agreed to be examined every two years. More than thirty years later the town has seen some changes, but the study is still going on and, it is a very important source of information about coronary heart disease.

The link between high blood pressure and coronary heart disease has been shown in several other studies besides the Framingham study. A similar study in Britain – the British Regional Heart Study – has shown that high blood pressure can double the risk of developing coronary heart disease.

Intervention studies have provided further evidence, showing that reducing blood pressure can reduce coronary heart disease rates. The MRFIT project in America and the North Karelia trial in Finland tried to reduce blood pressure as well as blood cholesterol levels in their 'special advice' groups and met with some success. The lower blood pressure levels may well have contributed to the fall in coronary heart disease rates in both studies.

In Europe, during the late 1970s, several countries collaborated on a project with the help of the World Health Organisation. Some 60,000 men aged from 40 to 50 were involved in the study and they were employed in 80 different factories in Belgium, Italy, Poland and the UK. Here, too, falls in blood pressure levels helped to reduce coronary heart disease rates, although in the UK coronary heart disease did not decline at all. The reason for the UK's poor performance seems to be that the efforts to persuade the men to change their habits were less vigorous here than they were in the other countries.

Once again, though, the story is not so simple. High blood pressure is very common in Japan, but Japan is famous, in the medical world, for its low rates of coronary heart disease. There are also countries with very similar levels of blood pressure but different rates of coronary heart disease.

Is blood pressure a likely cause?

When blood is pushed from the left side of the heart through the arteries the pressure has to be high enough for the blood to reach all parts of the body (see page 23). Although the arteries are tough and stretchy on the outside, the lining is very smooth and thin and if this delicate layer is damaged, cholesterol can start to build up. The arteries seem to be able to cope with the normal everyday ups and downs in blood pressure levels, but if blood pressure stays high the constant force of the blood through the arteries means they are more likely to be damaged.

Evidence from Japan actually supports the theory that high blood pressure causes damage to the arteries. Even though coronary heart disease rates are low in Japan the population has a serious problem with strokes. Strokes are caused by narrowed, blocked or damaged arteries in the brain, in the same way as coronary heart disease is due to damaged arteries in the heart.

Smoking

How strong is the link?

Another important risk factor for coronary heart disease is smoking. Major investigations such as the Framingham, and the British Regional Heart Study, show that smokers have two or three times the risk of developing coronary heart disease than non-smokers. The risk increases with the number of cigarettes smoked and the number of years during which someone smokes.

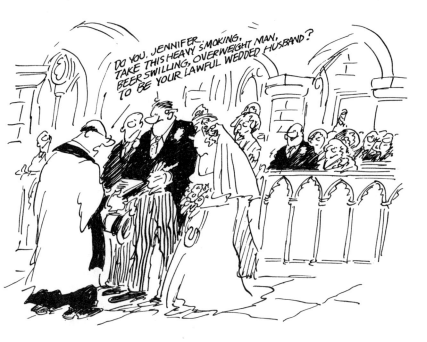

Further evidence was gathered from Richard Doll (see page 183) and Richard Peto's twenty-year study of British doctors, from 1951 to 1971. As well as demonstrating the strength of the link between smoking and coronary heart disease, this study also showed that doctors aged 45 or younger who were smokers had fifteen times the risk of a fatal heart attack compared to non-smoking colleagues of the same age.

Intervention studies bear out the theory that when people stop smoking they reduce their risk of coronary heart disease. MRFIT, the WHO collaborative project in Europe and the North Karelia project in Finland all link falls in smoking rates to a reduction in coronary heart disease rates. Many studies show that the risk falls quite rapidly as soon as a person stops smoking, so that five years after giving up smoking, an ex-smoker's risk is almost the same as that of a non-smoker. The results of the British Regional Heart Study, however, were not quite so encouraging and seem to show that the benefits of stopping smoking take longer. None the less, all the evidence points in the same direction: smoking is linked very closely to an increased risk of coronary heart disease and stopping smoking decreases that risk.

But even when the evidence seems so clear, there are some exceptions to the rule. The Japanese, for instance, are very heavy smokers and yet they do not have high rates of coronary heart disease. Smoking is very common in Mediterranean countries too and they also seem to be less susceptible to the consequences – at least in terms of coronary heart disease (although rates of lung cancer in these countries are rising).

Is smoking a likely cause?

In fact, smoking can quite easily be established as a cause rather than just a link. While cigarettes contain a mixture of about 4,000 chemicals, the two that are of particular interest in the coronary heart disease story are nicotine and carbon monoxide.

Nicotine is poisonous enough to be used as an insecticide in the garden and is as toxic as either cyanide or arsenic. It is also an addictive drug that makes parts of the brain react as if the person is under stress. Hormones such as adrenalin are released into the bloodstream, the arteries constrict, the heart beats faster (and so needs more oxygen for the extra work), the blood gets stickier and more likely to clot and there is a temporary rise in blood pressure. This rise in blood pressure, although temporary, may increase the risk of damage to the arteries and the likelihood of atherosclerosis developing. If the arteries have already become furred up with atheroma, then stickier blood might also create a clot that blocks one of the coronary arteries.

The carbon monoxide present in cigarettes can be just as dangerous as that in car exhaust fumes. Oxygen in the blood is carried by haemoglobin but, when carbon monoxide is present it combines with the haemoglobin, in competition with oxygen. This means that the blood is carrying less oxygen at a time that the heart needs more oxygen, due to the fact that the nicotine is making the heart work harder. Carbon monoxide, like nicotine, also seems to make the blood more likely to clot, increasing the risk of an artery becoming blocked.

The three major risk factors

Raised blood cholesterol, high blood pressure and smoking are the three major risk factors for coronary heart disease. The evidence shows (see page 183) that they are more likely to cause coronary heart disease than be linked merely by chance. It is clear that each risk factor on its own may not cause coronary heart disease, but the combination of any two or three of these risk factors can be significant for coronary heart disease. These risk factors multiply if present in any one of a number of combinations. For example, if you smoke you may have twice the risk of a non-smoker, and if you also have raised blood cholesterol your risk may rise to four times that of a non-smoker with lower blood cholesterol. But if you smoke *and* have raised blood cholesterol *and* have high blood pressure, then your risk may rise to *eight times* that of someone without any of these three risk factors. The diagram overleaf shows how the three main risk factors can combine to increase dramatically the chances of developing coronary heart disease.

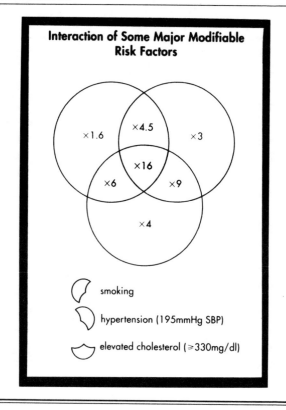

Interaction of Some Major Modifiable Risk Factors

×1.6 ×4.5 ×3

×16

×6 ×9

×4

smoking

hypertension (195mmHg SBP)

elevated cholesterol (≥330mg/dl)

CASE HISTORY OF A HEART ATTACK VICTIM

Eric has raised levels of cholesterol in his blood and athero-sclerosis begins. His arteries are being damaged by high blood pressure, so new fatty streaks are appearing and getting larger all the time. Each time Eric smokes his heart beats faster and needs more oxygen, but the coronary arteries cannot get the oxygen they need because the blood is carrying too much carbon monoxide instead. This is made worse because Eric's coronary arteries have been narrowed by plaques or lumps of atheroma and finally, because the smoking has made his blood stickier, a clot forms on one of the plaques and jams the artery. The blood supply to that part of the heart is cut off. Eric has a heart attack.

In the UK average levels of blood cholesterol in adults are 5.9 millimoles per litre (mmol/l) compared to the very low Japanese levels of around 3.8 mmol/l (see the section on cholesterol on page 57). High blood pressure is common in the British population and about one-third of British adults are smokers. Small wonder, then, that Britain has one of the worst rates of coronary heart disease in the world. Scotland and Northern Ireland have even higher rates than England and Wales. An English or Welsh man aged between 35 and 74 is twice as likely to die from coronary heart disease as an Italian man of the same age, three times more likely than a Frenchman and *eight* times more likely than a man in Japan.

Fibrinogen: the new risk factor?

Although raised blood cholesterol, high blood pressure and smoking appear to be the strongest risk factors, a number of other factors have also been linked to increased risk of coronary heart disease. One relative newcomer is fibrinogen. This protein in the blood is present when blood clots form, so it may prove to be critical in turning narrowed arteries into blocked ones. If this is so, then the more fibrinogen there is in the blood, the more likely it is that clots will form which might clog up the arteries.

A British GP, Maurice Stone, was one of the first people to notice the link between fibrinogen and an increased risk of coronary heart disease. A study at the Northwick Park Hospital in London has also found that higher levels of fibrinogen are linked to higher rates of coronary heart disease and this has also been supported by the Framingham study. Northwick Park has even shown that fibrinogen can be a more accurate predictor of coronary heart disease than blood cholesterol. Many more studies will need to be done before we can see if this risk factor answers the 'key questions' outlined on page 17.

Another difficulty with fibrinogen, at this early stage of research, is that it is very difficult to measure accurately and even the same individual's measurement can vary. Research into the role of fibrinogen is a promising area, but, as yet, it is too early to reach any conclusions on how to lower fibrinogen levels.

Overweight: the old risk factor?

People's image of the typical heart attack victim is often someone who is very overweight (obese, in medical terms). It is true that many studies, including the Framingham and the British Regional Heart Study (see page183), have shown a link between obesity and coronary heart disease. The picture is complicated by the fact that very overweight people also tend to have raised levels of blood cholesterol (with a higher proportion of the 'bad' LDL cholesterol and a lower proportion of the 'good' HDL cholesterol) and also high blood pressure.

By using various statistical techniques it is possible to calculate how much of the increased risk of coronary heart disease in overweight people is due to raised blood cholesterol, how much is due to high blood pressure and how much might be caused simply by being overweight. It seems that, once blood cholesterol and blood pressure have been taken out of the picture, being overweight doesn't in itself seem to add much to the increased risk. But, since being overweight seems to cause high blood pressure and raised cholesterol levels (and losing weight lowers both), being overweight is seen as a risk factor.

There is also growing evidence that it is not necessarily the weight which causes the problem, but where it goes. Men tend to put on weight round the belly – 'apple shaped' – whereas women are more likely to put weight on around the hips and thighs – 'pear shaped'. The risk of a heart attack from being apple rather than pear shaped seems to be more important than the total amount of extra weight gained (see also page 62). But smoking and alcohol both appear to exaggerate the pot-belly, perhaps by altering the way sex hormones are handled by the body.

Risk factors: the ones you can change and the ones you can't

There are a number of risk factors for coronary heart disease which, with the best will in the world, are impossible to change. They are age, gender, family history, ethnic group and diabetes.

Age

Part of the tragedy of coronary heart disease is that it can strike in the prime of life. But although coronary heart disease accounts for one in three of all deaths in men before the age of 65, most coronary deaths occur after 65. All the cohort studies (see page 13) show that deaths from coronary heart disease steadily increase with age.

But it is probably not age in itself which causes the problem. It is more likely that, over a lifetime, raised blood cholesterol coupled with high blood pressure and/or smoking take their toll, so that, with age the more likely it is that angina or a heart attack will result. Coronary heart disease is not, therefore, the inevitable consequence of getting older. And even if your first heart attack is after the age of 65, who is to say it is any less of a tragedy? It may not count as 'premature' in statistical terms but if you're not ready to go then it's premature for you!

Gender

Coronary heart disease is often thought of as a man's disease. It is true that more men than women die of it and if you compare men and women between the ages of 35 and 44, then a man is five or six times more likely to die from coronary heart disease than a woman. All the cohort studies show this strong link. But this evidence needs to be treated with a certain amount of caution, because it focuses on premature deaths from coronary heart disease and not illness or what happens after the age of 65.

Many studies of the risk factors involved in coronary heart disease have looked only at men. Some, like Framingham, have looked at both men and women but hardly any research has focused on women alone.

After cancer, coronary heart disease is the leading cause of premature death among women. And although women may not die from the disease, they are almost as likely as men of the same age to suffer from angina. After the menopause there is an increase in the death rate so that, after 65, coronary heart disease is the main cause of death for women and the rate is almost the same as for men over 65. Also, if a woman has heart surgery, it tends to be less successful because women's hearts and arteries are generally smaller and less easy to operate on than men's.

It seems likely that female hormones (particularly oestrogen) offer some protection against some aspects of coronary heart disease. Before the menopause women tend to have higher levels of 'good' HDL cholesterol in their blood, but it is not clear how, if at all, this might be linked to oestrogen levels. Women who have had an early menopause or who have had their ovaries removed experience a fall in oestrogen levels and their risk of coronary heart disease consequently rises. Conversely trials in the United States have shown that post-menopausal women who have oestrogen replacement therapy can reduce their coronary risk by up to 45 per cent. But if oestrogen is given to men (usually as a form of treatment for some other disease) their coronary risk seems to rise rather than fall. Perhaps the only lesson that can be learned at this stage is that prevention is just as important for women as it is for men.

The contraceptive pill

A number of studies have shown that taking the pill can increase blood pressure and blood cholesterol levels and make blood more likely to clot. These results must be treated with caution as modern pills tend to have lower doses of hormone than the ones involved in these early studies. It is also not clear whether the pill is a risk in itself or only if it affects blood pressure, blood cholesterol and clotting. None the less, the combination of raising three risk factors is a serious one.

For women on the pill, the key is to have regular check-ups. Your family planning clinic or GP should measure your blood pressure every time you go for new supplies. If there are any indications that blood pressure is rising, you may need further tests. The longer you have been on the pill the more likely it is that problems may develop. It is also vital to stop smoking. Any adverse effects from the pill will be multiplied by the effects of smoking. It may come down to a choice between smoking or carrying on with the pill. If you can't stop smoking you may be advised to change your method of contraception.

Family history and FH

There is a condition known as familial hyperlipidaemia (FH), the consequences of which further support the idea that raised blood cholesterol levels are a major cause of coronary heart disease. Because of a genetic abnormality which affects their liver, people with FH cannot get rid of the cholesterol in their blood very well. Consequently their blood cholesterol levels are very high indeed and their risk of developing coronary heart disease, even if their blood pressure is normal and they do not smoke, is very high. Around one person in 500 has this genetic problem and it is possible for FH sufferers as young as 20 to have heart problems. FH is a very particular problem requiring special care (the address of the association for FH sufferers is listed on page 186).

Many studies have also indicated that if your father or brother has a heart attack before the age of 50, or your mother or sister has a coronary before 55, then your own risk may double or even quadruple. No genetic explanation for this has yet been found. There seems to be no missing protective gene, and no particular gene which makes people more susceptible. There are probably combinations of genes that affect blood cholesterol, blood pressure and blood clotting, for example, but the possible permutations are endless. An equally likely explanation is that habits, as well as genes, run in families. So if parents smoke their children are more likely to smoke. If parents eat an unhealthy diet, their children probably will too. This theory has been backed up by findings in which people not genetically related, such as wives and husbands, have similar blood cholesterol and blood pressure levels.

Ethnic group

Very little research has been done as to whether some ethnic groups are more predisposed to coronary heart disease than others. Certainly, from all the studies that have been done around the world, no race or ethnic group seems to be immune to coronary heart disease. Even in Japan, where high blood pressure and heavy smoking are prevalent, coronary heart disease rates are low. It seems that it is low blood cholesterol levels, and not the fact that they are Japanese, that protects them. Japanese people who move to the United States very quickly start to acquire American levels of blood cholesterol and coronary heart disease.

There is one ethnic group, however, which does seem to be more prone to coronary heart disease. People from India, Sri Lanka, Pakistan and Bangladesh appear to have higher rates. Asians who have moved to South Africa, Trinidad, Singapore and the UK have all been found to have higher rates of coronary heart disease than the native South Africans, Trinidadians, etc.

There are very few indications as to what might cause higher rates of coronary heart disease in Asians. Smoking, raised blood cholesterol and high blood pressure have all been eliminated (by statistical techniques) from the explanation. New results seem to suggest that diabetes (see below) and body shape (i.e. being 'apple' rather than 'pear shaped') may be important factors. Clearly there needs to be much more research in this area.

Finally, there is one risk factor that seems to be linked to race and that is blood pressure. There are some places in the world where high blood pressure is unknown. Bushmen in the Kalahari, some tribes in the Congo and highlanders in New Guinea may face a number of difficulties in the modern world but they do not suffer from high blood pressure. Nor does their blood pressure rise with age, as seems to be the case in Western countries. On the other hand black people, particularly black women in America, have higher than average blood pressure. The stress of poverty and racism has been suggested as a possible cause, but when black and Causcasian (white) Americans in similar circumstances are compared, it is still the black Americans who suffer more from high blood pressure. No one knows why this is the case, nor if the same phenomenon occurs in Britain.

Diabetes

People with diabetes have problems controlling the level of sugar in their blood, which can lead to a range of disabling diseases and even death. One of the most common causes of death for diabetics is coronary heart disease. The Framingham study and a number of others showed that diabetics are more likely to suffer from heart failure and to die from coronary heart disease. Male diabetics may have double the risk of dying from a heart attack and female diabetics seem to be worse affected still, with three times the risk of coronary death of non-diabetics. Diabetics also seem to have a higher than average risk of developing other artery diseases, such as strokes and peripheral arterial disease (see page 32). Furthermore, Asian people in the UK are more likely to be diabetic and we have already seen that Asians seem to have a higher risk of coronary heart disease.

Does this mean that diabetes itself is a risk factor for coronary heart disease? The picture is far from clear. Some evidence from other parts of the world, for example the Pima Indians in the United States, shows high rates of diabetes but low rates of coronary heart disease. And there are complicating factors: diabetics, particularly those who develop the problem later in life, tend to be overweight and have raised blood cholesterol levels and high blood pressure. Some research also shows that diabetics have raised levels of fibrinogen in their blood, making it more likely to clot. If all these risk factors for coronary heart disease are taken out of the picture, the role of diabetes itself seems much smaller.

There is also the issue of the diet recommended for diabetics. Until about ten years ago, diabetics were advised to eat a high fat diet. We shall examine the links between a fatty diet and blood cholesterol in chapter six but it is probably true that this high fat diet increased diabetics' risk of developing coronary heart disease. For a number of reasons this advice has now changed and diabetics now eat a low-fat, high-fibre diet to help them control their blood sugar levels. This may mean that, in future, diabetics' coronary risk may be reduced.

Everything causes heart disease?

So far, following years of research, more than 200 factors have been linked to an increased risk of coronary heart disease. Snoring and soft water, for instance, have been associated with an increased risk, whilst sunshine and siestas have been linked to lower risks! The links between these minor risk factors and coronary heart disease are not very strong and need to be analysed by means of more research.

Some of these minor risk factors may prove to be important additional factors which, while not as important as blood cholesterol, blood pressure and smoking, could perhaps be avoided. So each time you read another 'shock' story in the papers about yet another new coronary heart disease risk, try to keep these key questions in mind: how strong is the link? and is it a likely cause? This is how the Coronary Prevention Group assesses new evidence, and until our expert advisers are satisfied, it is treated with caution.

CHAPTER 4

ARE *YOU* AT RISK?

GIVEN that there are a number of risk factors which can combine over a number of years to increase your chances of developing coronary heart disease and that many people in Britain have some of these risk factors – raised blood cholesterol levels, high blood pressure and smoking – so the average risk of developing coronary heart disease in this country is very high compared to other countries.

How many people in the UK actually have coronary heart disease?
The only statistic that can be used with any certainty is the number of deaths from coronary heart disease – currently it is over 170,000 each year. Many more people have the disease, but the signs of illness from coronary heart disease are not clear cut. The difficulty of diagnosing coronary heart disease means that it is hard to know how many people are suffering from the disease at any one point in time. Because the process of atherosclerosis is often silent it is also difficult to know how many people are at risk of developing coronary heart disease. But there are some tests which can give an indication of your personal level of risk. An isolated result from, for example, a blood cholesterol test, is insufficient information on which to base a diagnosis of coronary heart disease, or indeed for you to implement advice on coping with the disease. The results of each individual test need to be interpreted to take into account *all* the other risk factors. Without this assessment there is a danger that a single result may be unnecessarily worrying or falsely reassuring.

Blood cholesterol tests

Finding out about blood cholesterol levels in an individual used to be a very slow, complicated and expensive business involving laboratory analysis of blood samples. Nowadays it is possible to have the results in minutes. The machines which can do this analysis are compact enough to sit on a desk and need only a drop of blood (a pin-prick from your finger) to do the test. Unfortunately these machines cost several thousand pounds each and so are rare in doctors' surgeries. Some of the analysis is still very difficult, so laboratory tests are still used.

The easiest measurement for either a laboratory or a desk-top machine to make is the total amount of cholesterol in your blood. The most common scale of measurement in Britain is millimoles per litre of blood (mmol/l). A millimole is a measure of the number of molecules in the blood. Another scale, more common in America, uses milligrams per decilitre (shortened to mg/dl) and measures the weight of cholesterol (in thousandths of grams – milligrams) in every tenth of a litre (decilitre) of blood (mg/dl). To convert one to the other the formula is $1 \text{ mmol/l} = 38.7 \text{ mg/dl}$.

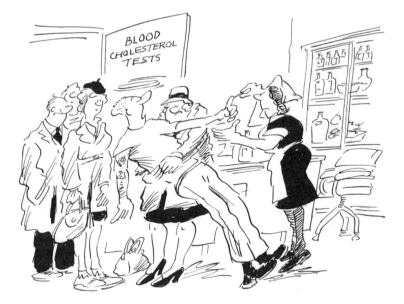

It is sometimes possible to see blood cholesterol levels. If an individual under 50 develops corneal arcus – a white circle round the edge of the iris (the coloured part of the eye) – it can indicate high levels of blood cholesterol. Small fatty lumps, or xanthomas, on the tendons at the back of the ankles and wrists, or xanthelasmas, fatty lumps on the eyelids, are two other signs in older people. But the only accurate way to measure blood cholesterol is to have a blood test.

A person with FH (the genetic tendency to have very high levels of blood cholesterol) may have a level of 11.0 mmol/l or more but the average level of blood cholesterol in the UK is 5.9 mmol/l. This looks fine, until it is compared to the Japanese average of only 3.8 mmol/l. Although Japanese levels of cholesterol would do wonders for the UK rates of coronary heart disease, it is widely agreed that it is rather an ambitious target to reduce levels to this extent. Instead there is broad international agreement that in Britain we should aim for a level of 5.2 mmol/l (or 200 mg/dl) or less.

This doesn't mean you should be very worried if your level is 5.3 mmol/l (or that you can heave a sigh of relief if it is 5.1 mmol/l). There is no 'cut-off' point below which you are fine and above which you are in the danger zone. An individual's blood cholesterol measurement varies from day to day and can be affected by that person's general state of health, the time of day or even the time of year (it seems to be higher, for example, in winter) and pregnancy. If you do decide you want a blood cholesterol test and your result is a fair amount higher than 5.2 mmol/l, it is worth having a second test to confirm the results. If the difference between the first and second measurement is larger than 1.0 mmol/l, a third test should be considered so that a more accurate average can be calculated.

It is also possible to test for different types of cholesterol in the blood. It has been seen that cholesterol carried by LDLs tends to stick to the artery walls and not the cholesterol carried by HDLs. There are also particles called very low density lipoproteins (VLDLs) and these are quite easy to measure (although for the test to be accurate you should not eat for 12 to 14 hours, or preferably overnight, with no breakfast before the test). The VLDLs carry a type of fat called triglyceride and this substance has also been linked to an increased risk of coronary heart disease.

Triglyceride levels tend to be higher in people who are very overweight, or who have an alcohol problem. Levels are also higher in diabetics and in women on the contraceptive pill. All these factors have also been linked to coronary heart disease. Disentangling the role of triglycerides from all these other factors has proved almost impossible so far. As triglycerides seem to be involved in the mechanism which makes blood clot, it is likely that there is some connection between triglycerides and coronary heart disease, but how the connection might work, and how important it might be, remains unclear. At present, if your triglyceride level is above 2.2 mmol/l your doctor will probably want to do a few more tests.

If your blood cholesterol test measures HDLs and triglycerides as well as the total, then it is possible to work out how much LDL there is in your blood. The formula is:

$$\text{LDL} = \text{Total cholesterol} - \text{HDL} - (\text{triglyceride} \div 2.19)$$

At the moment the level of LDLs is the most important indicator of your risk of coronary heart disease in terms of the cholesterol factor. Total cholesterol measurements are a good enough guide to the level of LDLs: if total cholesterol levels are high then LDLs will be too. The opposite is also true – low blood cholesterol levels usually indicate low LDL levels.

There is some dispute about how important HDLs are. The theory is that, since the HDLs' job is to take cholesterol away from the cells, the more HDLs you have the more of your cholesterol will be taken away instead of getting stuck to your artery walls. Some of the surveys, in Framingham and Finland, for example, have shown that higher levels of HDL do seem to offer some protection against coronary heart disease. More support for the theory comes from the fact that a woman's HDL levels tend to be higher than those of a man of a similar age and women's coronary death rates are lower than men's. The problem is that low HDL levels are so closely linked to other risk factors – such as being overweight, smoking and low total blood cholesterol – that it is difficult to tell if HDL levels are significant in their own right.

The most important fact to remember about blood cholesterol

testing is that it only tests *one* of the risk factors. A high reading does not mean you are about to have heart attack and a low reading does not mean you have nothing to worry about. All the other factors described in chapter three have to be taken into account too, so the test should be done by your doctor or another medically qualified person such as a nurse or dietitian. He or she will be able to balance the cholesterol measurement against all the other factors, assess your personal risk level and offer the appropriate advice and treatment if necessary.

Measuring blood pressure

Measuring blood pressure levels is much easier and cheaper than measuring blood cholesterol. It wasn't always the case though, and until around 1900 an artery had to be cut to measure the pressure. Around that time an Italian doctor invented the first blood pressure testing machine or sphygmomanometer, which could measure pressure without the need for surgery. The device consisted of a thin tube of mercury set against a millimetre scale, connected to a hollow rubber cuff and a bulb to inflate the cuff. The basic design is still the same today.

Air is pumped into the cuff, which is placed round the upper arm. The mercury rises up the scale. After a few seconds the air pressure in the cuff is high enough to squeeze the main artery in the arm so that the blood can't flow through. The air is slowly let out of the cuff while the doctor or nurse listens to the arteries through a stethoscope. After a couple more seconds the blood pressure is just high enough to force the artery open and the sound it makes can be heard in the stethoscope. At this point the level of mercury on the scale is noted. It is usually between 100 and 140 millimetres. This measurement shows blood pressure at its highest, when the heart beats and pumps blood through the arteries. The heartbeat is called systole (see page 23) so this measurement is the systolic pressure.

The cuff carries on deflating, with the artery now opening and closing and still making a noise that can be heard through the stethoscope. After a final few seconds the noise disappears because the artery stays open. The pressure in the cuff has fallen to the same level as the pressure in the arteries and the level of mercury on the scale is noted again. By now it is usually between 60 and 90 millimetres and it shows blood pressure at its lowest point, when the heart is resting between beats. This is called diastole so this measurement is the diastolic pressure.

So if you're told your blood pressure is 110/70, it means the systolic pressure measures 110 millimetres on the mercury scale and the diastolic pressure is 70 millimetres. Both numbers are well within the normal range although, like blood cholesterol, there is no cut-off point which marks where normal blood pressure begins and abnormal starts. So, for example, 130/85 is still within normal blood pressure ranges but would give that person a slightly higher risk than the individual with blood pressure of 110/70.

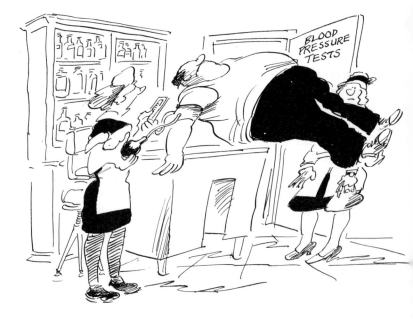

Blood pressure measurements are similar to blood cholesterol tests in several other ways. Firstly, levels can fluctuate in the same person. If you've just had a cigarette, or you're in a rush, or bursting to go to the toilet, or just nervous about having your blood pressure tested, your blood pressure will go up. But these are the temporary variations which don't increase your coronary risk. What matters is your resting blood pressure, so it's always a good idea to arrive early for your test and sit quietly for a few minutes.

Secondly, the first measurement shouldn't make you jump to conclusions. A result on the high side usually leads to another one or two tests, if only to make sure you weren't still nervous about the test. Thirdly, high blood pressure (or hypertension, in medical terms) is only one risk factor for coronary heart disease. As with blood cholesterol, all the other factors have to be considered alongside this measurement so 'normal' blood pressure alone doesn't mean you have a completely clean bill of health and hypertension doesn't mean you should get your will out of the attic.

Finally, high blood pressure usually has no symptoms. Like blood cholesterol there may be some signs – in the case of very high blood pressure, possibly headaches – but the only way to be sure is to get it checked. The Government now recommends that all adults have their blood pressure checked at least once every three years. It's cheap and simple to do and blood pressure is also a useful indicator of a number of other diseases besides coronary heart disease. Strokes in particular are very closely linked to high blood pressure and some kidney problems can also be picked up with a blood pressure test.

Sometimes you won't even need to make a special trip to have a blood pressure test; the medical staff in family planning clinics and blood donor centres, for example, routinely check their clients' blood pressure. It is also possible to buy blood pressure testing machines so you can measure your own levels at home. Unfortunately a recent survey by Consumers' Association showed that a selection of sphygmomanometers that were tested were found to be extremely unreliable and so could not be recommended for anyone wishing to measure his or her own blood pressure levels. But as you can ask your doctor or practice nurse to test it for you, there is no real need for this kind of DIY machine.

Are you overweight?

No special tests are needed to answer this question. All you need are weighing scales. There is a difference, though, between wanting to lose a few kilos because you feel it will make you look better, and being so overweight that it is a risk to your health. The chart below shows that you can be quite a lot heavier than a person the same height and still not put your health at risk. In fact, we have already seen that for coronary heart disease, it may be other factors associated with being overweight, such as raised blood cholesterol and high blood pressure, that are important and not being overweight in itself.

Far too many people, particularly women, make themselves thoroughly miserable by being constantly on different diets to try to lose quite small amounts of weight. It's beyond the scope of this book to examine the reasons for this but unless you're clearly in the 'fat' or 'very fat' section of the chart or your doctor advises it, there's no real need to lose weight for your heart's sake *if* all the other indicators are fine.

Having said that, being overweight is not irrelevant to coronary heart disease and recent research has shown that fat

Relationship of weight to height, defining the desirable range (0), and grades I, II and III (obesity)

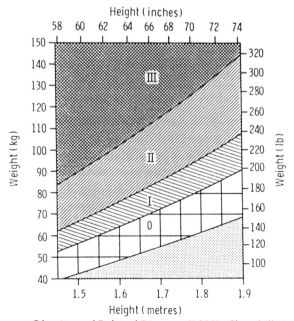

(From J Garrow, *Obesity and Related Diseases* (1988), Churchill Livingstone.)

around your middle may be worse than fat on your hips and thighs. So when your waist measurement is larger than your hip measurement it really is time to strip off the weight. But since it's easier to keep the flab at bay than to try and remove it once it's arrived, chapter six will take a look at how to stay in the 'OK' section of the chart.

Symptoms of coronary heart disease

For some people, staying perfectly healthy is no longer an option. For them, the symptoms of coronary heart disease have already started to show. By far the most common symptom is a gripping, squeezing pain in the centre of the chest. If the pain is brought on by exertion, anger, excitement or stress and disappears after a few moments' rest, it is an indicator of angina. That means the coronary arteries are probably furred up with atheroma and cannot supply enough oxygen to meet any extra demands on the heart. If the pain does not fade after a short time, say 10 to 15 minutes, then it is more likely to be a heart attack.

One problem with identifying the pain of coronary heart disease is that the intensity of the pain can vary enormously. It can be quite mild and feel a little like indigestion, so much so that some heart attack victims have taken indigestion tablets and ignored the pain. The other problem is that pain in the chest might actually *be* indigestion. Sometimes an overwhelmingly painful sensation can make you feel or even be, sick and look extremely pale.

Palpitations (see chapter two, page 36) might be a sign of coronary heart disease. A silent heart attack may have damaged the heart's own pacemaker, making it feel like it's racing, or going far too slowly. On the other hand, it may be a pacemaker problem that has nothing to do with coronary heart disease, or be one of those odd ectopic beats which don't seem to signify anything.

Even more confusing are symptoms which don't appear to come from the heart at all. Feeling breathless or extremely tired, for example, are common symptoms. This is not the kind of breathlessness brought on by playing squash or going for a brisk walk, but gasping for breath when you're doing something quite ordinary which doesn't normally have this effect on you. It may be that one or more silent heart attacks have weakened the heart muscle so that it can't pump properly. Blood might begin to back up into the lungs, making them congested and breathing difficult, or it may be that not enough oxygen-rich blood is reaching your muscles, leaving them tired and feeling heavy.

Otherwise these symptoms might result from a different problem altogether – heart valve trouble for example – or it may be simply that you are very tired and you need a good rest. Frequently, the symptoms we have briefly described may happen in combination. If you have any symptoms such as these or feel at all worried, the best solution is to visit your doctor.

Diagnosing coronary heart disease

Your doctor does not have any tricks that can instantly distinguish the pain of coronary heart disease from any other kind of pain. But GPs are very experienced in interpreting these symptoms in the light of your medical history (including risk factors such as whether or not you smoke and if any other family member has had heart trouble) and adding them to the results of a physical examination. All these facts will give your doctor a good idea of what might be wrong, but it is usually necessary to go through a few tests just to confirm the diagnosis.

A blood test, for example, can yield a range of useful information. Following a heart attack, certain chemicals are released by the damaged heart muscle into the blood and can remain there for several hours afterwards. If these chemicals are found, it can confirm that the pain you felt was a heart attack and not something unrelated to heart disease. Your doctor might also ask the laboratory to check your blood sugar levels, because it is possible to have a mild form of diabetes (now known as impaired glucose tolerance) without being aware of it. Later on the doctor might test your blood cholesterol levels since, although the results won't explain your symptoms, they can be a useful benchmark if you are trying to reduce your levels later on. The cholesterol test won't be done immediately because, if you have had a heart attack, it takes a few weeks for blood cholesterol levels to stabilise.

Electrocardiography

Electrocardiography (or ECG) is one of the most common tests used to confirm a diagnosis of coronary heart disease. Small metal or plastic discs (called electrodes) are taped to the chest, arms and legs where they can pick up the tiny electrical signals being sent from the pacemaker through the heart's atria and ventricles. The signals are sent down twelve leads connected to a machine which amplifies the signals and makes a trace on continuously moving paper.

The trace is called an electrocardiogram and it can show a range of heart diseases including rhythm problems, heart failure, or if part of the heart muscle has died following a heart attack. Unfortunately, the ECG may show 'abnormalities' even when the heart is perfectly healthy (a false positive result) or the reading can appear perfectly normal even though there may be quite serious heart disease (a false negative result). ECGs are particularly bad at confirming a diagnosis of angina, and up to 60 per cent of angina sufferers may have a normal ECG.

Stress test

Instead of an ordinary or 'resting' ECG, people with angina pain are often given a different type of ECG test – a stress or exercise ECG test. Exactly the same procedure is followed, except that instead of taking the measurements when the person is sitting quietly, the monitoring takes places while the person is walking on a treadmill or pedalling on a stationary cycle. Blood pressure measurements are also taken at various times during the test, which starts fairly gently and gets gradually more difficult.

The test can last for fifteen minutes, depending on the age and general state of health of the person being tested, and stops when the person becomes too tired, breathless, or feels in too much pain. But even if the person being tested feels fine, the medical staff running the test may stop it if there are any signs from the ECG or from the blood pressure measurements that all may not be well. Because it imitates the circumstances in which people may have an angina attack, the stress test is much more accurate than the resting ECG. Even so, it is not 100 per cent accurate and, for unknown reasons, this test cannot confirm coronary heart disease in women as easily as in men.

Heart scanning

Because of these accuracy problems, another test is sometimes added to the stress test and this is known, among other things, as heart scanning. This involves injecting a radioactive chemical – an isotope – into the bloodstream. The level of radioactivity is very small indeed and only lasts for a short time, so the risks are very low (though to be on the safe side the test would not be done if you were pregnant).

Once the isotopes reach the heart doctors can 'see' how the heart is behaving via a gamma camera close to the chest which picks up the radioactivity. Different isotopes can be used, depending on which part of the heart needs to be observed, and the tests sometimes adopt the name of the chosen isotope, for example a thallium scan. Heart scanning can show the extent of any heart damage and the position of blocked arteries and can be undertaken separately from the ECG if necessary.

One or a combination of the tests already described is usually sufficient to confirm your doctor's diagnosis, which may be that you have coronary heart disease or that your heart is fine. The following test is normally only done if surgery seems necessary.

Cardiac catheterisation and angiography

Although some types of heart surgery now seem quite commonplace, operating on the heart is still a delicate business and it is important to have the most accurate information possible before the operation takes place. In order to obtain such details a long, flexibile plastic tube (about the width of the tube inside a ball-point pen) is inserted into the main artery via the arm or leg. This tube, the catheter, is guided by X-ray, up to and even inside the heart. Attachments on the catheter can measure blood flow and blood pressure and can also detect problem valves. A dye that can be detected by X-ray can be injected into the heart through the catheter and the resulting X-ray image of the pumping chambers is called an angiogram.

It is also possible to position the catheter at the entrance to the main coronary arteries on the heart's surface and inject the dye into each of them. Any severely narrowed sections or blockages will show up clearly on the X-ray. This is called an arteriogram. This test rarely produces false positive or false negative results but there is always a very slight risk that the procedure will actually trigger a heart attack so it is never undertaken lightly.

It is also not a very comfortable test to undergo since although you will probably be sedated during the 30 minutes to an hour it takes to do the test you will still be awake. Although you won't feel the catheter itself moving about, you might feel a burning or flushing sensation when the dye is injected and have a headache and a nasty taste in your mouth for a while afterwards. On the other hand cardiac catheterisation is a good deal more comfortable than it used to be and some people can take their mind off the discomfort by watching the pictures of their own heart working.

Some of the tests we have not described here, such as echocardiography, are more useful in detecting other heart problems such as congenital heart disease. Others are simply new variations on old tests, made possible by computerisation and miniaturisation of technology. But new developments are progressing all the time and may help not only the diagnosis but also the future treatment of some forms of heart disease.

CHAPTER 5

WHAT YOU CAN DO – STOP SMOKING

IF YOU are a smoker, the simplest and most effective way to reduce your risk of developing coronary heart disease is to stop smoking. If you are over 20 and you don't smoke, the chances are that you never will: 90 per cent of smokers start before the age of 20. Most people have their first cigarette when they are very young. About one third of those people who become regular smokers have started before the age of 9. Almost 22 per cent of girls are regular smokers as early as 15 years old. One of the reasons why children begin to smoke is because their parents are smokers. Children are twice as likely to take up smoking if their parents do.

Smoking is now a minority habit: it is estimated that around a third of the UK adult population smoke. So smoking is still far too common, but that leaves two-thirds of the population at a potentially lower risk of coronary heart disease. And studies have shown that over half of all smokers want to give up. Over the last 15 years more than 10 million people have given up smoking. If you're a smoker considering giving up, it might be comforting to know that you're not alone in wanting to give up and that so many people have succeeded.

Many former smokers will tell you how easy it was for them to stop; that they did it first time, with no problems, and have never looked back. You might be like them. On the other hand, some people try unsuccessfully and stories such as these are discouraging to someone who wishes to give up. There are no magic cures or tips for instant success.

Why stop smoking?

The most powerful reasons for giving up smoking are for reasons of health. It has already been explained that a smoker carries double the risk of coronary heart disease of a non-smoker. If you have any of the other risk factors shown in the diagram on page 46, then your risks can multiply. To give you some idea of the scale of this risk, consider the following statistics: of 1,000 young men who smoke regularly, on average one will be murdered, six will be killed on the roads and 250 will be killed by tobacco-related diseases, a greater proportion of which will be by coronary heart disease.

Many other diseases have also been closely linked to smoking. They include strokes, peripheral arterial disease, cancer (of, for example, the lung, mouth, throat, bladder, pancreas, cervix and penis), bronchitis and emphysema. Smoking has also been linked to impotence in men and reduced fertility in women.

Is it really worth giving up?

If you're a smoker you may think that the damage has already been done. In terms of reducing your risk of coronary heart disease, and for many of the other diseases, the answer to this question 'Is it really worth giving up?' is a resounding 'yes!'. The benefits begin on day one. Without cigarettes the blood is absorbing oxygen instead of carbon monoxide so that your heart and the rest of your body is getting a better oxygen supply and your blood is less likely to clot. This means that your heart isn't under such a strain as when you smoked. Gradually your body will begin to return to normal and after a few years (the estimates vary but it could be as little as five years) your risk of developing heart disease will be almost the same as a non-smoker. The longer you have been a smoker and the more cigarettes you smoke, the longer it will take, but the greater benefit will be.

Extra motivation

Some people will get extra motivation for giving up by realising what they are doing to other people's health as well as their own. We have already mentioned, for example, that smokers' children are much more likely to smoke than the children of non-smokers. Smokers' children are also likely to suffer from the results of passive smoking which may include diseases such as bronchitis, pneumonia, asthma and glue ear.

Many women stop smoking when they become pregnant. Smoking during pregnancy can lead to smaller, less well developed babies, slower growth later in life, an increased risk of birth defects and, at worst, miscarriage or stillbirth.

Some people give up smoking because they have a close friend or relative who suffers from a disease such as bronchitis or asthma both of which are made worse by breathing in other people's tobacco smoke. It has been firmly established that passive smoking can increase your risk of developing lung diseases. The evidence is also growing that passive smoking can even lead to coronary heart disease and it is likely that passive smoking can be damaging to people who already have coronary heart disease.

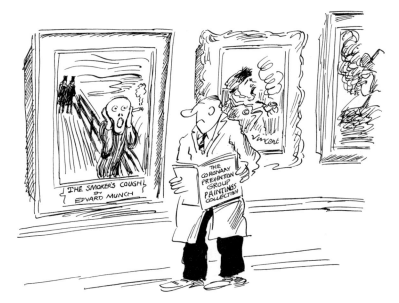

In some ways, concern about your own health is the best psychological condition for success. The danger in stopping for someone else is that if they are no longer there, you slip back into your old habit.

For some people though, knowing about the personal health risks of smoking just isn't enough. Particularly if you are a young smoker, ill-health may seem many years away. But there are more immediate benefits to giving up smoking and perhaps the most persuasive is the extra money you'll save. In 1991, an average packet of cigarettes costs £1.80. If you are an average smoker, at 20 a day, then your habit is costing you over £12 every week, or over £54 each month and over £650 for a year. You'll also need to take into account extras such as matches or lighters, plus extra cleaning costs for the ash and cigarette butts in your home, and extra decoration costs to cover the tar stains which have built up on your paintwork and wallpaper.

Other immediate benefits of stopping smoking include the effect on your appearance. Your clothes, hair, breath and mouth no longer smell and, since smoking speeds up the wrinkling and ageing of the skin, this process slows down again after giving up. Violent coughing fits first thing in the morning will disappear too, though, for some people, the first few weeks can produce a feeling of tightness in the chest and *worse* coughing fits. This does *not* mean giving up smoking is bad for you: this is just your body's way of getting rid of some of the 'gunge' that has built up in your lungs. You may also find you get a sore throat for a short while. This is because smoking simultaneously irritates and numbs your throat. When you stop smoking the numbness wears off before the irritated throat has recovered. Many successful ex-smokers report feeling more 'aware'. Their sense of taste returns and their senses in general feel clearer and sharper. Many people also feel much more confident and full of life. Make no mistake – taking control of your life and deciding not to smoke can be exhilarating.

Any one of the reasons outlined above might be enough to convince you that now is the time to stop smoking. Whatever the reason or combination of reasons, a personal conviction that you really *want* to stop smoking is best. If there is any magic ingredient to stopping smoking successfully it is that you must be utterly convinced that you want to stop.

Risks attached to giving up: fact and fiction

'I'll get fat'

By far the most common reason suggested for not giving up smoking is the fear of getting fat. Some people even suggest that putting on weight is as bad, if not worse, for your health than smoking. Very overweight people do tend to have raised blood cholesterol levels, high blood pressure and are more prone to develop diabetes. All these factors are linked to an increased risk of coronary heart disease.

But it has been calculated that to increase your risk to that of smoking twenty cigarettes a day, you would have to gain around 10 stones (about 64 kilos) in weight. The average weight gain for someone who gives up smoking is about four pounds (two kilos) and even this is usually temporary.

There are several reasons why you might gain weight if you give up smoking. First, smoking can interfere with your digestive system so that you don't absorb the energy (calories) from your food properly. (This doesn't mean that smoking makes you slim. One American study showed that the fattest women were the heaviest smokers.) So even if you don't eat more after you stop smoking you may gain a little weight because your body is using food more efficiently. Second, smoking can suppress your appetite, so when you stop you may actually feel hungrier. Third, smoking can dull your taste buds so that when you've given up, food actually tastes better so you might want to eat more.

These are all *possible* effects; they are not inevitable and many people do not put on an ounce of weight when they give up smoking. In fact you could make stopping smoking just one part of your 'health campaign' and take the opportunity to change your diet at the same time. There are several advantages to this, not least that changing your diet might remove some of the 'triggers' to having a cigarette.

'I'm too stressed – I need cigarettes to relax'

Dealing with stress is a complicated business and hundreds of books have been written on the effects of stress and how to cope. Not a single expert on stress recommends smoking as an effective way to relax. Cigarettes don't make the cause of your stress disappear. And if you look around you and compare smokers with non-smokers, you can see that smokers, if anything, sometimes appear more stressed, not more relaxed. So why do smokers *feel* more relaxed?

What you crave when you're under stress and reach for a cigarette is nicotine. There is evidence that stress can increase the rate your body breaks down nicotine, leading nicotine levels to fall and triggering the craving. So when you have a cigarette, your body is simply getting a temporary 'fix'. Until the vicious circle of craving nicotine is broken, you will never be free to relax properly.

Worse still, cigarettes can produce effects that mimic some of the effects of the body in a state of stress. So, for example, the heart rate increases, adrenalin is released into the bloodstream and blood pressure rises. The effects of stress will be discussed in more detail in chapter eight, but if you're feeling stressed your heart rate will already be higher, with adrenalin coursing through your blood and your blood pressure raised. Having a cigarette makes all of this worse.

How to do it: going it alone?

By far the simplest method of giving up is to go 'cold turkey' and just do it. Millions of people have stopped smoking without special help. If you have never tried to give up before, it's worth trying 'cold turkey' first, because if it works for you, you're free in one simple step.

If it doesn't work the first time, mix your own unique combination of methods until you find one that works. Giving up smoking is a very personal affair and the suggestions here are simply a selection of some of the common methods which have been known to work.

The big build up

You might have some difficulty with going 'cold turkey'. For example, you might find the withdrawal symptoms surprisingly difficult to cope with if you're not expecting them. Being irritable, finding it hard to concentrate and having cravings for nicotine are by far the most common symptoms and if you've been a very heavy smoker for many years, you may find them quite severe. On the other hand, you may be like thousands of others who sailed through giving up without the slightest sign.

If you've tried to stop before and you know you get withdrawal symptoms it is important to plan how you're going to cope. Any of the following suggestions might help: time each craving (so you can see how they get shorter and less frequent); take ten slow, deep breaths and concentrate on your main reason or reasons for giving up; go for a walk (or cycle, or jog, or swim – whatever's convenient so long as it's active); have an apple (or a piece of sugar-free chewing gum, or chew a liquorice stick); clean your teeth (your mouth will feel fresh, so you won't want to spoil it with a cigarette).

Some methods of stopping smoking recommend keeping a smoking diary for a week or more to find out what kind of smoker you are (e.g. habitual, liking the handling and paraphernalia of smoking, psychological 'addict'), to count how many you actually smoke, and to spot which are your most and least important cigarettes of the day. Opinions vary as to whether you should give up the most important first or the least important first and some people will find the process of keeping a diary more difficult than giving up. In the end, the most important cigarette to give up is the first one of the day!

People also vary in their views about publicising their own process of giving up. Some find that the more people know, the better. Every friend and relative can be a source of moral support and some people feel that if they tell enough people it will be too embarrassing to start smoking again. Others say that it is just one more pressure thay can do without and prefer a private battle with the weed. Either way, make a solemn vow for the day you're going to stop, to underline the seriousness of your commitment. Written down or in your head, public knowledge or silent promise, the contract is a binding agreement with yourself to give it your best shot.

Keep a record of how well you are doing too. Perhaps the best way is to save all the money you would have spent on cigarettes then treat yourself to something you will enjoy at the end of the first week or month or even a year.

Finally, think carefully about how you're going to deal with those situations in which you *always* have a cigarette. If your favourite time is just after you've finished your meal, for example, don't just sit there – go and wash up! If you like a cigarette with a cup of coffee, drink tea, or fruit juice or something else instead. If you like a cigarette with alcohol it might be worth avoiding an alcoholic drink for the first week or so – a few drinks can play havoc with your willpower. If someone offers you a cigarette don't say, 'I'm giving up', say, 'I don't smoke.' It's more positive and doesn't give that person the opportunity to tempt you away from your choice.

But if you do have a moment of weakness, for whatever reason, and have a cigarette, don't despair. Whatever you do, don't give up and smoke as normal for the rest of the day, promising to start again tomorrow. Try to think about how you could tackle the situation differently next time. Would it be better to avoid that situation altogether for a while? Rethink and have another go.

Join a group

All of the above techniques (and more) can be used and developed in a 'stop smoking' group. Many people find that such groups can provide the knowledge, skills and mutual support that giving up alone can't match. They are being set up all over the country. 'Stop smoking' groups vary enormously in their approach, but usually entail five to eight sessions of one or two hours each and will probably be led by someone trained in counselling and motivation techniques. Very often the group leader will also be an ex-smoker. The groups also vary in price, from commercial rates to a nominal charge or even free, depending on circumstances. If this method appeals to you, your main problem is likely to be finding a group. The addresses listed on page 186 include organisations that should be able to help with this. At the end of the day, you could always set one up yourself.

Herbal remedies and other helpful hints

There is quite a range of products on the market which extravagantly claim that they can help you to stop smoking. None of them is a miracle cure but some of them may help boost your resolve. However, none of them will give you resolve if you lack it.

Nicotine chewing gum

By far the best researched of these aids is nicotine chewing gum. Because it contains a small quantity of nicotine it can help reduce withdrawal symptoms in people who suffer particularly badly from them. If you feel that craving or irritability is hampering your attempts to stop, this product might be a useful aid. Nicotine gum is less dangerous than smoking since it doesn't contain carbon monoxide (or the tars which cause cancer) and its effectiveness is improved if it's combined with a 'stop smoking' course or counselling.

There are other preparations on the market containing nicotine which work on the same principle as nicotine chewing gum but these have not been as thoroughly tested.

Other aids do not contain nicotine, but aim to ease withdrawal symptoms using other ingredients. Some herbal remedies available in health food shops and by mail order also work on this principle and it is not clear how, if at all, these ingredients might work.

'Dummy' cigarettes

Some smokers find that it is not nicotine withdrawal symptoms that bother them but having nothing to do with their hands. To tackle this aspect, a number of types of dummy cigarettes have been developed which imitate the look and feel of a cigarette, but which don't burn at all (menthol and similar ingredients are substituted so that when you inhale you get a cool sensation in your mouth). The problem here is that people find that the dummies are too reminiscent of the real thing and they are tempted to go back to smoking. Playing with a pencil, doing puzzles, learning origami and knitting are just some of the other things you could do with your hands!

Two other 'aids' should not really be considered as such at all, since they are in many respects no safer than smoking. Special filters added to cigarettes can trap some of the tar and nicotine as you inhale, but there is a tendency for smokers to inhale more deeply and frequently to compensate for this reduction, cancelling out any benefit that there might have been. Herbal cigarettes, although they do not contain nicotine, still produce carbon monoxide (and tar) so they are no safer than ordinary cigarettes.

Pipes, cigars and low-tar cigarettes are not classified by the medical profession as aids to stopping smoking, but some smokers do find them helpful. Lifelong pipe and cigar smokers are at lower risk of coronary heart disease than cigarette smokers because they tend not to inhale deeply. However, their risk is not zero and the risk of developing some cancers, for example lip cancer, is the same as for cigarette smokers. Those who turn to pipes or cigars to wean themselves off cigarettes, do tend to inhale, and so increase their coronary risk. Similarly, with low-tar cigarettes, smokers may simply inhale more often and more deeply in order to maintain their nicotine levels. This can increase the levels of carbon monoxide and actually increase the coronary heart disease risk.

Alternative therapies

Finally, a number of alternative therapies are available. Acupuncturists sometimes insert a staple into your ear and you press it if you feel a craving for a cigarette. However, not all acupuncturists agree that this is an appropriate use for their particular skill. If you want to try acupuncture, do make sure you go to a properly qualified practitioner (see page 187 for the address of the governing body).

Aversion therapy works on the principle that if smoking can be made revolting enough, you will never be able to face a cigarette again. Techniques include chain-smoking until you're almost sick and mild electric shocks each time you inhale. As these methods are potentially dangerous, particularly if you have an existing illness, it is not advisable to try DIY aversion therapy. There is, unfortunately, no association to control standards in this field.

All of these therapies may have varying degrees of success but most of them are likely to work out a little expensive. A personal recommendation is worth considering, but what works for a friend will not necessarily work for you. Certainly, if you've tried everything else it is worth trying the harmless therapies.

Research seems to show that, with the possible exception of nicotine chewing gum, no single aid to stopping smoking is more effective than another. Personal advice from your GP, on the other hand, does seem to be quite effective – perhaps because he or she is talking about your individual risk and not the risks of smoking in general. But, ultimately, there really is no substitute for willpower.

CHAPTER 6

WHAT YOU CAN DO – EAT A HEALTHY DIET

MANY of the important risk factors for coronary heart disease already looked at – blood cholesterol levels, blood pressure, blood clotting – can be affected by what we eat and drink. This section will look at each of the main nutrients in our diet and assess the benefit of changing it. It will also examine the research which has been done linking some types of drinks to coronary heart disease and will look at some of the 'miracle' dietary supplements which have recently appeared on the market.

Saturated fat

Links with blood cholesterol

Ancel Keys' study of seven countries (see page 12) was one of the first (and is still one of the most respected) studies showing the link between blood cholesterol and coronary heart disease. Keys' research also showed a strong link between the amount of saturated fat consumed in each country and the average level of blood cholesterol. The higher the proportion of saturated fat in the diet, the higher the blood cholesterol levels were and, consequently, the higher the rates of coronary disease. In another study Ancel Keys showed that every person in a group of volunteers who was fed a diet high in saturated fat increased his or her level of blood cholesterol.

The same links have been found in a range of other research projects; a major study of civil servants in London (the Whitehall study), a survey of employees of the Western Electric

Company in Chicago and research in California all showed that saturated fat consumption was closely linked to blood cholesterol levels and coronary heart disease rates.

More evidence has been added from intervention studies and two of these studies were particularly interesting. Because coronary heart disease has been linked to so many risk factors (it is a multifactoral disease), most efforts to reduce people's risks have been directed towards reducing all the risk factors at once. The theory is that the greater the extent to which risk factors are reduced, the sharper the fall in coronary heart disease rates will be. However, two intervention studies have focused on just one risk factor – blood cholesterol – and attempted to reduce it by reducing the amount of saturated fat in the diet.

The Los Angeles Veterans study looked at 846 American military veterans aged 54 to 88. The men were split into two groups and for the next eight years one group was given a low saturated fat diet. The special diet group had fewer heart attacks and fewer deaths from heart attacks than the control group, with the younger veterans (under 65), on the low fat diet, doing best of all. A similar study was done in Finland in two mental hospitals, where some 700 men and 600 women were studied for a total of 12 years. Again, those people who had been in the group following a low saturated fat diet showed less coronary heart disease than those following the normal Finnish diet.

Despite these and other convincing research results, it has been much more difficult to show the saturated fat and blood cholesterol link *within* populations than it has *between* populations. There are a number of possible reasons for this. First, there is the problem of collecting the information. There are established methods of estimating the diet in each country in order to compare the countries. Agricultural production figures, plus imported food figures, minus exported food figures (and anything eaten by animals) give a broad indication of what people in the country are eating. Provided the same methods are used for each country, a reasonably accurate comparison will be obtained.

The problem with looking at groups of people within a country is that accurate information is difficult to gather. The main method of finding out what people eat is to ask them, but people's memories are notoriously unreliable. There are more sophisticated and expensive techniques, of course, including asking people to keep a record of what they eat each day and taking blood and urine samples, which can sometimes show how much of a particular nutrient has been eaten. But the problem of getting accurate information about individuals' diets remains.

Second, there is the problem of timescale. Scientific research is an expensive business and it is possible only rarely to keep surveys going for more than four or five years. If you are doing an intervention study, you hope to see changes in the group in which you are 'intervening' and not in the control group. But to expect changes after four or five years of intervention, when the risks of coronary heart disease may take 40 or 50 years to build up is perhaps expecting too much.

Despite these difficulties, saturated fat has been shown to have a strong link with blood cholesterol levels. The one Nobel prize ever awarded for research into coronary heart disease was given to Joseph Goldstein and Michael Brown, the scientists who discovered that saturated fat interferes with the ability of the liver to deal with cholesterol.

Research with animals has underlined the point. A diet high in saturated fat raises blood cholesterol levels, furs up the arteries and increases the risk of coronary heart disease in animals. The reverse has also been shown to be true: a low saturated fat diet in animals can lower blood cholesterol levels, reversing the process of atherosclerosis and reducing coronary risk.

Reducing saturated fat intake

The message is clear: eat less saturated fat. In theory, it is possible to eat no saturated fat at all, and still remain healthy, since the body doesn't need it. In some places in the world saturated fat accounts for as little as 3 per cent of the energy (calories) in the diet. In the UK saturated fat accounts for around 17 per cent of the energy (calories) in the diet, and in Scotland, where men have the worst rates of coronary heart disease in the world, it reaches 20 per cent.

In practice, though, it would be impossible to eat no saturated fat at all. The fat in all kinds of food is always a combination of three types: saturated, polyunsaturated and monounsaturated fats. The fat in food is usually made up of mainly one kind of fat, with the other two making up the balance. So, for example, 100 grams of butter contain 49 grams of saturated fat, 26 grams of monounsaturated fat and 2 grams of polyunsaturated fat (this doesn't add up to 100 grams because butter contains other nutrients as well as water).

This imbalance in the composition of the fat in food makes it easier to recognise which foods contain which type of fat. Foods which are high in saturated fat, for instance, are usually solid at room temperature, whereas polyunsaturated oils tend to be liquid. Dairy products are composed of mainly saturated fat and they account for some 42 per cent of the saturated fat in the UK diet. Meat and meat products are also prime sources of saturated fat, taking up another 22 per cent of the total, followed by

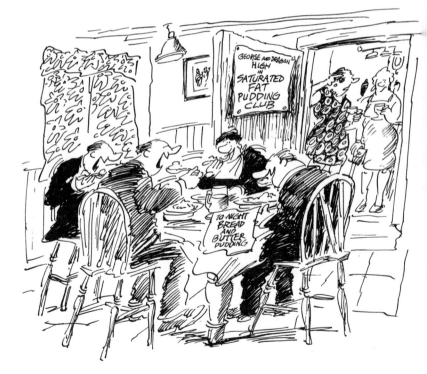

margarine, lard and other fats and oils at 19 per cent. The rest of the British saturated fat total comes from biscuits, cakes, chocolate, crisps, pastries and the like.

Does this mean the end for cheese sandwiches? Certainly not! Although simply eating less of the types of food listed above is by far the simplest way to reduce the saturated fat content in your diet, it is by no means the only way. Dairy products now come in a range of full-fat, medium-fat and low-fat versions, so it is much easier than it used to be to continue to eat dairy products without bumping up your saturated fat intake. A pint of semi-skimmed milk, for instance, has a mere 5.6 grams of saturated fat compared to 14 grams for ordinary milk and it tastes virtually the same. If you're a cheese lover, savour the full-fat types, (such as Stilton, and Cheddar occasionally) and choose lower-fat versions (such as Edam or cottage cheese) for everyday use. Butter fans who can't bear the taste of margarine and low-fat spreads just need to spread it more thinly (in New Zealand, where they are very serious about butter, all fridges have 'butter-softening' compartments so it can be spread sparingly straight from the fridge). Cream (of any type) should be enjoyed in moderation.

The meat industry, like the dairy industry, has responded to the challenge of healthy eating and developed leaner cuts of meat. Unfortunately meat *products* are less of a bargain for the health-conscious shopper. Meat pies and sausages alone account for around 9 per cent of the saturated fat in the British diet. As much as 27 per cent of the energy (calories) in a pork pie comes from the saturated fat in the meat filling and the pastry. In some ways it's easy to see why meat products contain so much saturated fat. Fat is much cheaper than meat and (with modern technology, plus colourings and flavourings) it can easily be disguised to look like meat in products such as pâtés, sausages, burgers and some chopped and shaped meats.

Even though chicken without the skin is a good low-saturated fat alternative to red meat, modern production methods seem to be increasing the level of fat in poultry to the point where, if the skin is left on, it can be fattier than some lean cuts of red meat. Chicken products often include the skin and are covered in breadcrumbs or batter. This means that they will absorb more fat if fried. A similar problem arises with fish products. Fresh or frozen fish is an excellent food, but when turned into fish cakes or fish fingers it contains more water and also batter to soak up the fat. If these are the family favourites, they should be grilled, not fried.

It is always better to grill rather than fry food, but when using cooking oils, fats and margarines, choose those that are labelled 'high in polyunsaturates' and use sparingly. Products labelled in this way are also relatively low in saturated fat (even though the label might not say so). An advantage of the soft margarines and low-fat spreads is that, as well as containing less saturated fat, they are easier to spread thinly, so that you can eat even less saturated fat.

Biscuits, cakes and chocolates contain a lot of saturated fat and sugar and because they are so tasty it's far too easy to eat a lot of saturated fat without realising it. Two chocolate digestive biscuits, for example, contain 4 grams of saturated fat, more than a chicken and salad sandwich!

Target levels

It is estimated that in Britain we should be reducing our saturated fat intake from the current 17 per cent to no more than 10 per cent of the energy (calories) in our food. For an average adult this means eating less than 20 to 30 grams of saturated fat each day. Trying to find out how much saturated fat you are currently eating could be an interesting exercise. Have a look for the nutritional information on any packets of food you have and see whether the saturated fat content is given. If a figure appears at all, it will be expressed as a number of grams per 100 grams of the product. It may also give you the number of grams in the actual weight of the product (which probably isn't 100 grams) and it *might* say how many grams of saturated fat you would get in an average portion of the product. There may be no nutritional information at all, or the information may only give the total amount of fat, not just saturated fat. There might even be a 'flash' on the front saying 'low fat', but the product may still not list the amount of saturated fat – the most important for reducing your heart disease risk.

However, the list of ingredients might give you some clues.

All foods have to list ingredients in weight order, so the main ingredient is listed first, followed by the next weightiest ingredient and so on. If you spot one or more of the following ingredients high up the list, the products is likely to be high in saturated fat: hydrogenated vegetable oil or fat, palm oil, cocoa butter, shortening, coconut oil, animal (beef/pork/chicken) fat, milk solids, non-milk fat.

Some vegetable oils (palm and coconut) also contain saturated fat. You should also be aware that 'hydrogenated' refers to a process in which unsaturated fats are turned into saturated ones.

Polyunsaturated fats

Polyunsaturates are an essential part of the diet – they are sometimes called essential oils or fats because, unlike saturated fat, the body cannot make enough for its needs. There is some evidence that, unlike saturated fat, polyunsaturated fat can actually reduce cholesterol levels. Although Keys' Seven Countries' Study showed a close link between saturated fat consumption and blood cholesterol levels and coronary heart disease rates, the link was shown to be even closer if polyunsaturates were also taken into account.

A number of theories have been suggested which might explain how polyunsaturates can lower blood cholesterol levels. It may be simply that the polyunsaturates are replacing the saturated fat and that this helps to reduce blood cholesterol levels.

Some doubts have been expressed about the benefit of polyunsaturates, in that there is a tendency for them to encourage the production of chemicals in the body called 'free radicals'. Some researchers think that these free radicals can damage the lining of the arteries, so leaving them more susceptible to atherosclerosis. Free radicals can be dealt with in the body by other chemicals called 'anti-oxidants'. Certain vitamins – A, C and E – are natural anti-oxidants. Fortunately, polyunsaturates have their own supply of vitamins, and vitamin A is often added to food products by manufacturers. There is therefore no need to eliminate polyunsaturates from the diet because of worries about the effect of free radicals.

Target levels of polyunsaturates

There are two different types of polyunsaturates: those from the seeds of plants (e.g. sunflower oil), called omega 6 or n–6 and those from fish oil, called omega 3 or n–3.

There have been more studies on fish oils than on plant oils. As far back as the 1950s a nutritionist called Hugh Sinclair drew attention to the possible benefits of oily fish in the diet. Research efforts were revived in the 1970s when a study noted that despite having similar amounts of fat in the diet, the Eskimos and the Danes had very different rates of coronary heart disease. The Eskimos, with a very large proportion of their diet coming from oily fish, had very low rates of coronary heart disease. Other surveys noted that, not only did the Japanese eat a lot of fish, but that Japanese fishermen (who ate even more fish) had even lower rates of coronary heart disease than the already low Japanese average.

Ancel Keys' survey did not support his view. Yugoslavians in his survey ate very little fish and had low rates of coronary heart disease. The Finns, on the other hand, ate a great deal of fish, but had one of the highest rates of coronary heart disease in the world (until they improved their record and were replaced by the UK at the top of the league table). But the Finnish diet contains a lot of saturated fat and the Yugoslavian diet very little. Any protective effect from the fish in the Finnish diet may have been overwhelmed by the saturated fat.

So it has not been conclusively proved that the omega 3 polyunsaturates found in oily fish protect against coronary heart disease. A number of theories have been put forward which might explain how fish oils work: for example, fish oil has been shown to make blood less likely to clot. Several studies have found that fish oils also reduce triglycerides in the blood (see page 57). But triglycerides may not be an important risk factor in coronary heart disease. Some research has shown that large amounts of fish oil can reduce 'bad' LDL cholesterol but also reduce levels of 'good' HDL cholesterol at the same time. Smaller amounts of fish oil even seem to increase blood cholesterol levels slightly.

Both types of polyunsatures together make up around 6 per

cent of the energy (calories) of the British diet. It appears that there is nowhere in the world where omega 6 polyunsaturates (from plant sources only) make up more than 7 per cent of the diet. Considering that fish is already an established part of the human diet the world over and the beneficial effect of omega 3 polyunsaturates (found in fish oil), intake could be increased by eating more oily fish. The following table lists types of fish that are good sources of omega 3 oils.

This table shows the type and amounts of fat found in a range of fish and shellfish.

Type of Fish	Grams of fat per 100g		
	Omega 3s	Saturated	Total
Smoked mackerel	3.3	4.1	15.5
Steamed salmon	2.9	3.4	13.0
Sardines tinned in tomato sauce	2.9	3.3	11.6
Grilled herring	2.8	2.7	13.0
Boiled crab	2.0	0.7	5.2
Baked kipper	1.9	2.3	11.4
Tinned salmon	1.8	2.1	8.2
Pilchards tinned in tomato sauce	1.5	1.7	5.4
Steamed trout	0.9	1.1	4.5
Steamed plaice	0.4	0.3	1.9
Steamed cod	0.3	0.2	0.9
Steamed haddock	0.3	0.2	0.8
Boiled prawns	0.2	0.3	1.8
Tuna tinned in brine	0.2	0.3	1.0
Tinned crab	0.2	0.1	0.9

This table has been adapted from data supplied by the Nuffield Laboratories of Comparative Medicine.

Try to include some of these types of fish in your diet two or three times a week. If you don't like fresh fish, there are plenty of alternatives in frozen packs and in tins (buy the type tinned in brine not oil or be sure to drain off all the oil). If you don't like any of the fish in the table, white fish or any other kind of fish is nutritious. Even if other types of fish are not particularly high in omega 3s, they are low in saturated fat (provided you don't fry in batter) and high in vitamins and minerals.

Monounsaturated fat

For a long time monounsaturates have been regarded as insignifcant in the coronary heart disease story. Recently, however, there has been a resurgence of interest in how the Mediterranean diet might protect against coronary heart disease. Some studies have suggested that olive oil (which is high in monounsaturates) may help to explain why the populations of France, Italy, Greece and their Mediterranean neighbours have much lower rates of coronary heart disease than the northern Europeans.

Critics have pointed out that the Mediterranean diet differs in many respects from a nothern European diet in that, for example, it includes less saturated fat and a higher proportion of fruit and vegetables, factors which may account for the differences in coronary heart disease rates.

So what is the consumer to make of this? Fortunately, there is no need to change the amount of monounsaturated fat in the British diet. Some 15 per cent of our energy (calories) already comes from monounsaturates and, since international experts recommend levels of between 10 to 15 per cent, this is one target that has already been met.

Total fat

All the different types of fat looked at so far have one thing in common: every gram of fat has 9 calories. This is more than twice as much as gram of carbohydrate or protein (which have around 4 calories per gram). If you eat a lot of fat of any kind, you are more likely to get fat. The average intake of fat in the UK is around 100 grams a day – about 38 per cent of our total calorie intake. Small wonder then that a recent survey showed that 45 per cent of men and 36 per cent of women are overweight, an increase of around 13 per cent over the last ten years.

International expert committees recommend that total fat intake should account for no more than 30 per cent of the total number of calories in the average diet – that means between 60 to 80 grams of fat a day (the lower figure is for women because they tend to eat less than men). This looks fairly low until you realise that most of the world's population thrives on 20 to 30 grams a day and in China less than 10 per cent of the energy (calories) in the diet comes from fat.

Cutting down on the amount of fat in the diet will help to stop the gradual increase in weight that with age seems almost inevitable in this and other Western countries. Although being overweight may not be linked directly to coronary heart disease, it is certainly associated with raised blood cholesterol levels, high blood pressure, high triglyceride levels and diabetes. As most of the fat in the British diet is saturated fat, cutting down on total fat is also a rough-and-ready way of reducing your saturated fat intake. And if you are already overweight, eating less fat will help you to lose fat.

Are there any risks attached to reducing fat intake?

From time to time there are stories in the papers which imply that it is dangerous or irresponsible to suggest that people should reduce the amount of fat, particularly saturated fat, in their diet.

One recent report claimed to have discovered that a low fat diet makes you less intelligent. In fact, the story behind the news was far less convincing. A researcher had noticed a link between people eating certain kinds of foods and the speed of their reactions to a type of test. High fat foods seemed to speed up reaction times and sugary foods seemed to slow them down. Scientists remain puzzled by this phenomenon. None the less, reaction times were linked to 'intelligence' – which was turned into the headline 'Fried breakfast can boost your brainpower'!

A more serious worry has been the link between low blood cholesterol levels and cancer. A number of studies have been looked at again and their data scanned for new information (a procedure called 'data-snooping'). An association has been discovered between some cancers and low blood cholesterol levels, but it is not clear if the low cholesterol levels are causing the cancer, or if the cancer is causing the low cholesterol levels. Certainly, none of the data has been able to show that a low fat diet led to low cholesterol levels, which in turn led to cancer.

International surveys would suggest exactly the opposite. In countries with a low average level of blood cholesterol, cancer rates are low. Other studies have linked high fat diets to increased rates of cancer. Saturated fat, in particular, has been associated with increased risks of breast and colon cancer. The evidence connecting high fat diets with cancer is not as strong as the evidence on fats and coronary heart disease, but it is certainly stronger than the statistical association between cancer and low blood cholesterol levels. So, far from being a risk, a low fat diet may reduce the risks of coronary heart disease *and* cancer.

The same data snooping also revealed a connection between low cholesterol levels and deaths from a number of unrelated causes, such as accidents, murder and suicide. This, too, was covered by a number of newspaper reports that interpreted the results as meaning a low fat diet made you so depressed you either killed yourself or someone else! In fact, the research showed a link between low blood cholesterol levels and violent deaths and not between low fat diets and these events. As we have seen, low blood cholesterol levels may sometimes be caused by some other factor (perhaps cancer).

There are bound to be other stories like this in the future. When you see them, remember the three key questions:

- How strong is the link?
- Is it a likely cause?
- What are the risks and benefits if I change my habits as a result of this evidence?

Coronary heart disease is such a complicated disease that we may never have absolute proof of its causes. What we *can* do is prove beyond reasonable doubt that the fats in your diet affect your risk of coronary heart disease and that it is more of a risk to ignore this than it is to change what you do.

Dietary cholesterol

It is actually quite difficult to study the effects of dietary cholesterol on blood cholesterol levels because cholesterol tends to be in the same foods which are high in saturated fat e.g. meat and dairy products. So if you are eating a diet which is high in saturated fat, you will also be eating a fair amount of dietary cholesterol.

However, there are some foods which are low in fat and saturated fat, but are high in dietary cholesterol. Liver, for example, is low in fat but high in dietary cholesterol since, as in humans, an animal's liver is where its blood cholesterol is processed. Other forms of offal are also high in dietary cholesterol. Shellfish with legs tend to contain more cholesterol, so shrimps, prawns and lobster have more than scallops, cockles and oysters. Egg yolks are perhaps the most common source of dietary cholesterol.

A person's blood cholesterol levels will rise if he or she eats plenty of cholesterol-rich foods such as eggs and prawns. But the effect is not nearly as powerful as that of eating saturated fat. Some individuals are more sensitive to dietary cholesterol than others and people with FH (familial hyperlipidaemia) have to be particularly careful. If you know your blood cholesterol levels are on the high side, you should save cholesterol-rich foods for special occasions.

The average intake of dietary cholesterol for a person living in the UK is about 400 milligrams. This compares to about 40,000 milligrams (or 40 grams) of saturated fat. If you are already following the suggestions for cutting your saturated fat intake to 20 to 30 grams, then your dietary cholesterol will automatically fall to the 300 milligrams or less which is recommended by international experts (unless you have a passion for shrimps, liver and eggs). Your liver makes around 70 per cent of the cholesterol your body needs, so lack of dietary cholesterol should not be a problem.

A recent survey showed that 41 per cent of people believed that avoiding cholesterol in the diet was the best way to reduce blood cholesterol. Only 36 per cent said that reducing the amount of saturated fat in the diet was important in lowering blood cholesterol levels.

The confusion in the minds of the public surrounding diet and cholesterol is probably because a diet low in saturated fat is often called a 'cholesterol-lowering diet' because that is what it *does*, and a diet low in dietary cholesterol is sometimes called a 'low cholesterol diet' because that is what it *is*. If you want to, or need to, be careful about dietary cholesterol, then you can reduce your intake of saturated fat as well. But a 'low cholesterol diet' on its own is not enough to lower your blood cholesterol levels.

So the first golden rule of healthy eating to remember is:

- eat less fat, particularly saturated fat.

You may remember a different type of advice about healthy eating and may be sceptical about this apparent U-turn in scientific opinion. In the post-war years people were urged to eat plenty of meat, milk, eggs and cheese – remember 'drinka pinta milka day' and 'go to work on an egg'? Current dietary advice appears to be the exact opposite. In fact, it's not so much the advice which has changed, but the nature of the public health problem. After the Second World War (and indeed before that) undernutrition was a major problem, leading to small, underdeveloped children who in turn became sickly adults. To boost growth nutritionists recommended protein-rich foods (such as meat and cheese) and, to fuel the growth, plenty of energy (calorie) -rich food. Gram for gram, fat has the most calories, so food such as meat, milk and cheese which are high in protein *and* fat were a double bonus.

This advice worked very well indeed and in time British children were no longer spindly specimens but became taller and heavier. Unfortunately, this advice was carried into adulthood and they became heavier adults too, with all the health problems that being overweight can entail. Only gradually, as evidence of a new public health problem – coronary heart disease – began to accumulate, did nutritionists begin to see the risks as well as the benefits of the high fat, high protein diet and revise it accordingly.

Complex carbohydrates

Complex carbohydrates are made up of simple sugars, starch and fibre. Few studies have been undertaken to investigate the role of starch in coronary heart disease and even fibre and sugar have not been as extensively researched as fats. None the less, some evidence does exist, particularly on fibre.

Fibre

Research in Puerto Rico, California and a study of London bankers showed a link between diets high in fibre and lower rates of coronary heart disease. Seventh Day Adventists (who are vegetarians and therefore have a high fibre intake) also have lower heart disease rates, even after taking into consideration the fact that they never smoke.

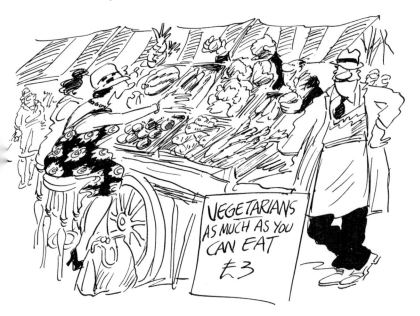

But a high fibre diet is often associated with a low intake of fat and saturated fat and it may be this which is responsible for the reduced coronary risk. There are also two different types of fibre, each having its own particular effect on coronary heart disease.

Insoluble fibre   is thought to have the least effect. It used to be called 'roughage' and provides much of the bulk of complex carbohydrates. It is found in, for example, the skin of fruit and vegetables and the outer husk of cereals. This type of fibre can certainly contribute to a healthy diet by making you feel full and so less likely to overeat. Insoluble fibre does not seem to have a direct effect on coronary heart disease.

Soluble fibre, on the other hand, may help to reduce blood cholesterol levels. It is found in fruits such as apples and oranges, leafy vegetables such as spinach and cabbage, beans and peas of all kinds and oats. Soluble fibre can be digested by chemicals, called enzymes, in the gut. The fibre tends to bind itself to other substances in the gut, such as bile acids, which contain cholesterol. The theory is that if cholesterol is bound to the soluble fibre, it cannot be absorbed and laid down on the walls of the arteries. The soluble fibre carries the cholesterol through the blood and eventually it is excreted. There are also some indications that soluble fibre may reduce the amount of fibrinogen in the blood, so making blood clots less likely.

Research into this theory is still in its early stages. Other scientists have produced results which show that soluble fibre is simply replacing the saturated fat in the diet and it is this factor which is responsible for producing the fall in blood cholesterol levels.

Increasing your fibre intake

Current UK fibre intake (both soluble and insoluble) amounts to 20 grams a day. Current scientific consensus (though not necessarily based on coronary heart disease research alone) recommends at least 30 grams a day and preferably more. Since soluble and insoluble fibre tend to be found in similar foods it is easy to increase your intake of both. They are contained in all kinds of fresh fruit and vegetables, all kinds of beans and peas, (not just baked beans and garden peas, but sweetcorn, kidney beans, chick peas, black-eyed beans, lentils and broad beans), all kinds of cereals, including bread, rice, pasta (particularly with the fibre left in) and breakfast cereals (though watch out for the hidden sugar and salt in some types).

The latest report from the World Health Organisation suggests that you should aim to have two pieces of fruit every day, plus a large portion of green leafy vegetable, a generous helping of another type of vegetable, plenty of potatoes and some salad. If this sounds a lot, bear in mind that you will have to cut down on the amount of fat in your diet and, unless you are on a weight-reducing diet, you will need to replace the calories with something else.

Fat can be replaced with large amounts of complex carbohydrates, which will not affect your weight. Remember, though, not to add fat to these foods. Fruit can be eaten without cream, salad vegetables don't need dollops of fatty mayonnaise, potatoes are better in their skins not in the chip pan and fresh vegetables can do without butter.

Are there risks attached to a high fibre diet?

Given that the evidence linking increased fibre intake to reduced risk of coronary heart disease is in its early stages, isn't this advice a bit premature? There are no known health disadvantages to a diet rich in complex carbohydrates. Whereas less than half of the UK diet consists of complex carbohydrates, most of the world population does very well on a diet that provides 70 per cent or more of its energy (calories) from this type of food.

The main drawback of such a diet for people who are not used to it is wind. Once your digestive system has adapted, though, this should not be a problem. Another possible drawback is that too much fibre can stop effective absorption of vitamins and minerals by the gut. However, this is more likely to happen if fibre is added artificially to the diet (in bran supplements, for instance). If fibre is eaten as nature intended, i.e. within the food in which it grew, vitamins and minerals should be plentiful.

There are other advantages to a diet rich in complex carbohydrates. Constipation would become a rare disorder and the risk of diabetes and some forms of cancer (such as bowel cancer) would also be reduced. So golden rule number two is:

- eat more complex carbohydrates.

Sugar

Sugar is also a form of carbohydrate, but it is a simple one. When complex carbohydrates are processed and refined they tend to lose their fibre and often become more sugary. This makes them easier to eat, and this is their 'fatal attraction'. Take an apple, for example. A whole apple contains fibre, starch, sugar and water. All the plant cells are intact and the sugar is inside the cell walls; this is called intrinsic sugar. In other words, the sugar is still inside the plant in which it grew.

An apple is quite filling and to eat two, three or four of them all in one go would be quite difficult. If you peel and core an apple, chop it up and boil it, you destroy most of the fibre and get rid of some water. Some of the sugar is now outside the cells which once contained it; this is known as extrinsic sugar. Eating an apple purée made of four or five apples wouldn't be too difficult, but it would be very hard to eat the same amount of calories in terms of whole apples. If you then make the apple purée into apple juice, the fibre disappears and almost all of the apple sugar is now extrinsic sugar. You could probably drink the juice of ten or more apples without feeling in the slightest bit full – ten times as many calories as a single apple in a few gulps.

This is not to say you shouldn't drink apple juice, or indeed any other kind of fruit juice. The example illustrates the point that it's very easy to eat too much extrinsic sugar without even noticing.

Sugar is not linked directly to coronary heart disease risk, but it may increase the risk of becoming overweight, which in turn can lead to raised blood cholesterol and triglyceride levels, high blood pressure and diabetes.

Another problem with sugar, though, is that it is often in the same foods as fat and saturated fat. Sugar and fat are both cheap ingredients, so mixing both together with a few flavourings and colourings produces all kinds of biscuits, chocolates and cakes. Combining fat, at 9 calories per gram, with sugar, which contains the easiest calories to eat without noticing, is a sure recipe for overeating. The UK is one of the largest consumers of these products in the world, for example, we eat our way through over 10 kilos (23 pounds) of biscuits per person per year.

Even without fat, extrinsic sugar is a poor type of food. Taken out of the plant cells, the sugar loses many of the vitamins and minerals it once had. Nutritionists often refer to sugar as 'empty calories', meaning that it is all calories and little else.

Cutting down your sugar intake

Cutting out sugar in drinks and on breakfast cereals is a good start. It probably isn't a good idea to replace sugar with artificial sweeteners because there are continuing doubts about the safety of chemicals used in them. It also doesn't help to re-educate your taste buds in this way: evidence suggests that people tend to use artificial sweeteners as well as and not instead of sugar. In fact, sales of artificial sweeteners have rocketed in the last few years, but sugar consumption has stayed almost exactly the same.

The other way to cut down on sugar is to eat fewer processed foods. Obvious examples of this type of food are biscuits, cakes and chocolate as well as sweets and sugary drinks. But sugar can turn up in the most surprising places. Foods with a healthy image, such as yoghurt and breakfast cereals, can contain the equivalent of several large spoonfuls of sugar. Finding this out involves careful checking of the label, as the manufacturers are most unlikely to admit to adding sugar in the nutrition information on the label. Sugar is usually hidden under 'carbohydrates', so that you can't tell if it's the type you want to eat – complex carbohydrates – or the type you want to avoid – simple carbohydrates i.e. sugar.

As with fat, the ingredients list (because it has to be there by law) can be helpful if you know what you're looking for; sucrose, dextrose, fructose, lactose, maltose, invert sugar, syrup and caramel are all forms of extrinsic sugar. The higher up the list of ingredients they are, and the greater the quantity, the more sugary the product is likely to be. Molasses, honey and brown sugar are not much different to plain white sugar.

Are there risks attached to cutting down on sugar?

It is a widely held belief that sugar is needed to provide the body with energy. But, in fact, the body eventually turns *all* the food that is eaten into energy. The occasions when you might need 'instant' energy are incredibly rare (and, in any case, your body holds emergency stores). Even people who have the most extreme need for energy, such as marathon runners, eat foods such as pasta, not chocolate bars, before a big race.

There are, however, a lot of other benefits besides the possibility of indirectly reducing your risk of coronary heart disease. The more sugar you eat and the more frequently you eat it, the more likely you are to suffer from tooth decay. If you eat less sugar your teeth will benefit. If you eat less sugar you are also likely to replace it with more nutritious foods. This can be very important for older people who tend to have smaller appetites since, although they don't need as much food, they *do* need as many if not more vitamins and minerals. If older people eat too many sugary foods they are not likely to be getting all the vitamins and minerals they need.

Golden rule number three is:

- eat less sugar.

Salt

Salt, like sugar, is not directly associated with an increased risk of coronary heart disease. It is, however, linked with a major risk factor – high blood pressure. Every country in which the population has a high intake of salt also has high average levels of blood pressure. Countries in which the population has a low salt intake have no such problems with blood pressure levels.

There is fairly firm research evidence to show that individuals suffering from high blood pressure (hypertension) need fewer drugs to control the condition if they also reduce their salt intake. Vegetarians, who also tend to eat less salt, have also been found to have lower blood pressure. But, as usual, there are factors which confuse the issue.

Salt is similar to sugar in another way in that it is a cheap ingredient which is often combined with fat to enhance its flavour. Sausages, pies and pâtés are good examples of this practice. Salt is often added to nuts, and crisps are a good example of a vegetable disguised with fat and salt. There are also fatty products which are traditionally salty such as bacon, ham, salami, smoked meat and fish, and most cheeses.

Could it be, then, that it is the fat and not the salt which is causing the high blood pressure? It seems likely that salt itself encourages the body to retain too much fluid. This increases the volume of blood in the system and the heart has to work harder to pump the blood round. Research also seems to show that too much salt (i.e. sodium chloride) upsets the delicate balance of minerals in the body. Potassium, magnesium and calcium are other minerals which have been linked to high blood pressure, but it is a lack of these elements rather than an excess which seems to be the problem.

Cutting down your salt intake

The only clear answer which has emerged is that some individuals are more sensitive to the effects of salt than others. So what should you do? Current UK levels of salt consumption are between 10 to 20 grams daily. Since the human body only needs 1 or 2 grams per days there is plenty of scope for cutting down. A reasonable target to aim for would be around 5 or 6 grams. The simplest way to achieve this would be to reduce the amount of salt added in cooking and at the table. Salt tends to mask the taste of food rather than enhance it so that, once you have got used to the true flavours, you will probably find that heavily salted food is quite unpleasant.

For this reason it is probably not worth spending a lot of money on salt substitutes. A better solution is to re-train your taste buds. The main problem is that, even though you've reduced the amount of salt you use at home, you're faced with the fact that 80 per cent or more of the salt in your diet is already in the food when you buy it.

Tinned fish and vegetables often contain far too much salt, but many manufacturers are now producing reduced salt or no-salt versions of their products. Butter can also be bought unsalted. Look out for other types of sodium on the label too. Monosodium glutamate (a flavour enhancer) is probably the most common, but other examples include sodium bicarbonate (baking powder) and some preservatives such as sodium benzoate, sodium nitrite and sodium sulphite.

Are there risks attached to cutting down on salt?

Will you suffer from lack of salt if you follow these guidelines? Lack of salt can lead to cramps and feeling very weak and feeble. But only in the most extreme conditions (e.g. working near a bakers' oven in a heatwave, or working extremely hard in a mine) do you need extra salt. If you're eating a healthy diet with plenty of fresh fruit and vegetables, you'll automatically get all the minerals you need, including sodium. Other benefits of a low salt diet might include a reduced risk of stomach cancer, since there is some evidence linking salty, smoked and pickled foods with this disease. Golden rule number four is:

- eat less salt.

Vitamins in fruit and vegetables

There has been little research into the effect of vitamins on the development of coronary heart disease but new findings have linked a high intake of fresh fruit and vegetables (which are rich in vitamins and minerals) to a lower coronary risk. It is difficult to know whether it is the fibre in fruit and vegetables which is responsible for this, or the vitamins and minerals, or both.

From research into polyunsaturates we know that certain vitamins (A, C and E) help to counteract any free radical chemicals in the bloodstream, making them less likely to damage the delicate lining of the arteries. Research into the causes of high blood pressure has indicated that minerals such as potassium may help to prevent blood pressure rising, or help to control if it is already high. Since fruit and vegetables are good sources of these free radical neutralisers and the minerals that regulate blood pressure, there are at least two possible ways (in addition to the beneficial effect of the fibre content) for these foods to help lower the risk of coronary heart disease. It seems likely, then, that the high consumption of fruit and vegetables by vegetarians may be one of the reasons why their rates of coronary heart disease tend to be lower than average.

You may be worried about eating more fresh fruit and vegetables because of the dangers of pesticides and other residues. But the risks to human health from chemical residues on fruit and vegetables is very small compared to the advantages of eating more of these foods. The use of pesticides, herbicides and other agricultural chemicals is controlled by a wide range of national and international rules and regulations and there should be few, if any, residues left on your food by the time it reaches you. To be on the safe side, it is always advisable to wash fruit and vegetables thoroughly before eating them. Many consumers are now turning to organic produce because of concerns about the use of pesticides, but organic fruit and vegetables are still much more expensive than their chemically treated counterparts. In time, and if demand continues to increase, then the prices of organic fruit and vegetables should begin to fall within the reach of more consumers. The other alternative is to grow your own produce.

Supplements

In recent years a number of products have begun to appear which make more or less outrageous claims about their ability to prevent coronary heart disease. You may think that, since there are laws to prevent manufacturers misleading the public about their product, then these claims must be true. However, for many years supplements have fallen into a grey area between laws which affect food, and laws which control drugs. The laws have now been changed to bring supplements firmly under the regulations which control food, but it is too early to say whether this will make it any easier to enforce high standards in this area.

Fish oil capsules

Although the evidence linking oily fish in the diet to the prevention of coronary heart disease (see page 89) has not been conclusively proven, the early indications are that increasing the amount of fish in a healthy diet offers far more benefits than risks. Some manufacturers of fish oil capsules have taken this as *carte blanche* for promoting their products as a miracle cure for coronary heart disease.

If your doctor has recommended that you take fish oil capsules (probably for the high levels of triglycerides in your blood), he or she will be using fish oil as a drug in your treatment programme. This programme will probably include advice on all the other risk factors. Any side effects from the fish oil, or any other drugs, will be carefully monitored and adjustments made to the dose accordingly.

This is quite a different matter to buying fish oil capsules yourself from a shop. Although there is little evidence of any harm (except to your bank balance) at low doses, fish oil capsules simply have not been in existence long enough for anyone to know what the long-term effects might be. And at low doses the evidence seems to suggest that they are not beneficial either. In any event, taking fish oil capsules as a *substitute* for lowering other risk factors, such as stopping smoking or eating a healthier diet, is completely ineffective.

Garlic tablets

Interest in the Mediterranean diet has focused mainly on the high intake of monounsaturates (in olive oil) and high consumption of fresh fruit and vegetables. Some research has also examined whether the Mediterranean habit of eating plenty of garlic might help to protect against coronary heart disease. There is some evidence that the chemical components of garlic, which give it its characteristic aroma, are also responsible for making the blood less sticky and so less likely to clot. Other evidence has not supported this view.

Certainly, if you like garlic in your food, there is no reason why you should not continue to use it, but the weight of research at the moment does not justify using garlic capsules or tablets. In any case, many of these products have removed the smell, the very element which might be doing some good.

Niacin

Like fish oil capsules, niacin may be prescribed by your doctor as part of your treatment for coronary heart disease. At the recommended doses between 100 milligrams and 300 milligrams a day, niacin should only be used under medical supervision. The recommended daily amount in food is a mere 15 to 18 milligrams a day and if you're eating plenty of wholegrain cereals (bread, rice and pasta) you'll be getting more than enough. Despite this, niacin capsules are available in some shops and there have been cases of people accidentally overdosing. Even at safe levels niacin can cause an unpleasant flushing or burning sensation and at high levels the liver may be damaged.

Vitamin tablets

If you are eating a healthy and varied diet there is no need to take vitamin tablets. Some people think that if vitamins are good for you then more vitamins must be even better. This is not the case. The body can only use so much of a vitamin, so any excess is usually flushed out. (Some research has even shown that the outer coating of some vitamin tablets is too hard for the body to digest so the tablets actually come out, intact, at the other end.)

At worst, you may be putting your life at risk if you take very high levels of vitamin tablets. Some vitamins can be poisonous at high levels and in recent years there have been a very small number of deaths due to overdoses of vitamin A. If, for any reason, you are not eating properly and feel that you may be missing out on your normal vitamin and mineral intake, ask your doctor or ask to be referred to a dietitian who will be able to advise you on safe levels.

Oat bran

Some shops are now selling oat bran as a supplement to sprinkle on your food or include in your cooking. Oat bran contains a lot of soluble fibre, which is thought to have a beneficial effect on blood cholesterol levels (see page 96). Eating foods which contain soluble fibre, such as fruit and vegetables, beans and peas and also oats, has several benefits and no obvious drawbacks. Adding oat bran to an unhealthy diet is more or less useless.

Coffee

A number of studies, particularly in Scandinavia, have shown a link between coffee drinking and blood cholesterol levels. Others, such as the large scale survey in Framingham, have found no such link. Since drinking coffee is closely associated with smoking, it has been difficult to isolate the effect of coffee itself but recent research seems to indicate that it is the method of making the coffee which is the key.

In Scandinavian countries coffee grounds are usually boiled and the resulting strong, black mixture is drunk unfiltered. Drinking this type of coffee does seem to raise blood cholesterol levels. Instant or filtered coffee doesn't seem to have the same effect, even though it still contains caffeine. Tea also contains a significant amount of caffeine and, luckily for the British, research so far has shown no link between tea drinking and coronary heart disease.

So there's little evidence to suggest that you should throw away the coffee machine, although there are other reasons why you may want to cut down. Coffee may have such a strong association with smoking that if you're trying to give it up it would be better to drink something else, at least for a while. Some people also find that coffee triggers odd (ectopic) beats and, since coffee is a stimulant, it also raises blood pressure levels (but only temporarily). If you are troubled by odd heart beats or high blood pressure it might be better to cut down your coffee intake.

Alcohol

Most studies have shown that people who drink a lot of alcohol have a higher risk of developing coronary heart disease. Alcohol consumption has also been linked to a number of coronary risk factors. High blood pressure is a common result of drinking too much alcohol. Since alcohol contains 7 calories per gram (second only to fat), increased consumption often leads to weight problems. Heavy drinkers are also more likely to be heavy smokers.

One study, however, showed that in countries where red wine consumption was high, coronary heart disease rates were low. These were Mediterranean countries and we have already seen how low saturated fat and high fibre consumption may contribute to the low coronary rates in these countries.

A number of recent studies have shown that non-drinkers had slightly higher rates of coronary heart disease than very moderate drinkers. Based on this, many people concluded that drinking alcohol is good for you.

However, a group of non-drinkers can be a mixture of lifelong teetotallers, ex-alcoholics and people who have given up alcohol due to some illness. It is likely that people from these last two groups have higher rates of coronary heart disease than the first group.

An increase in alcohol intake seems to have a beneficial effect on levels of 'good' HDL cholesterol. Unfortunately this seems to take effect only at a very high intake of alcohol, so that this marginal benefit would be more than cancelled out by the resulting higher blood pressure, increased weight and increased triglyceride levels, making the blood stickier.

There is no strong evidence to show that drinkers should take the pledge, so long as alcohol intake is moderate. Moderate means no more than two or three units of alcohol a day. A unit of alcohol is the equivalent of half a pint of ordinary strength beer or lager, a glass of wine, a single measure of spirit or small glass of sherry.

For women the levels are lower – no more than one or two units a day – because women tend to be smaller and have less fluid in their bodies. This lower fluid level means the alcohol is less diluted than it is in the average man.

Two units of alcohol a day is an upper limit, not a recommendation. You don't have to drink alcohol every day and you certainly can't save up your 'allowance' and drink it all on one day. Fourteen units or more of alcohol in one day is alcohol abuse and that way lies cirrhosis of the liver, some forms of cancer, brain damage, strokes and other forms of heart disease such as rhythm problems and cardiomyopathy (see page 37).

Summing up

The golden rules for a healthy diet can be summed up in four lines:

- eat less fat, particularly saturated fat
- eat more complex carbohydrates
- eat less sugar
- eat less salt

Translating this into the kinds of food to eat is just as simple:

- eat plenty of cereals – bread, rice and pasta – preferably the wholegrain versions with the fibre left in, and eat lots of beans and peas
- eat as much fresh fruit and as many vegetables as you like
- eat fish, poultry and unprocessed meat

CHAPTER 7

WHAT YOU CAN DO – EXERCISE

FOR many years the evidence has been accumulating to show that regular exercise can prevent coronary heart disease. The earliest study was by Jerry Morris who, in the late 1940s and 1950s compared the health of thousands of London bus drivers with that of bus conductors. He found that the drivers, sitting in the cab all day, suffered far more heart attacks than the conductors, whose job involved running up and down the stairs. Twenty years on, Jerry Morris and his team of researchers began a more ambitious survey, this time of around 18,000 middle-aged male civil servants working in an office. The research lasted ten years and showed that the men who took vigorous exercise at least twice a week in their leisure time had less than *half* the heart attacks and coronary deaths of the otherwise comparable, but less active civil servants.

Similar research was started in the USA and Ralph Paffenbarger's twenty-year study of dockers in San Francisco showed that those in physically active work had less coronary heart disease than their workmates doing lighter jobs. At the other end of the scale Ralph Paffenbarger also studied graduates from Harvard, one of America's most prestigious universities. He found that graduates who took regular exercise had less coronary heart disease than graduates who had opted for a more inactive life. But he also noticed that those who had been keen athletes at college did not seem to benefit from this youthful activity if they didn't keep it going in adulthood. The ones who hadn't been athletic at college had just as low rates of coronary heart disease as the college athletes, provided they took regular exercise when they left college.

Some 50 other studies have underlined these findings. However, a study of lumberjacks living in Finland in the 1960s showed that they had very high rates of coronary heart disease even though they had active jobs. Exercise, then, won't make you immune to effects of smoking and an unhealthy diet, although it does reduce these effects.

It has been found that on average people who exercise seem to smoke less, eat a healthier diet and are less likely to be overweight, and for a while it was thought that these factors, and not exercise, were protecting these people against coronary heart disease. But with statistical techniques it has been possible to take all these factors into account: exercise has emerged as a clear and important element in any strategy to prevent coronary heart disease.

There is still some debate as to exactly how vigorous and precisely how frequent exercise has to be before it starts to reduce coronary risk. Some evidence leans towards moderate exercise as being sufficient, whilst other results show that quite vigorous effort is required. The main point is that the exercise has to be more energetic than is usual for *you*. As for frequency, some scientists say 'every day', others say 'twice a week'. Researchers seem to agree that around 20 to 30 minutes of vigorous activity, two or three times a week is beneficial. All agree that this level of activity must be maintained regularly.

Beneficial effects of exercise

There is also a good deal of agreement about how exercise helps to reduce coronary heart disease. Exercise has been found to produce beneficial effects on all three major risk factors. First, it can reduce the total amount of cholesterol in the blood and, although the fall is not dramatic, it reduced the 'bad' LDL cholesterol more than the 'good' HDL cholesterol. So exercise can help to slow down the process of atherosclerosis.

Second, although it is not clear how it works, exercise has been shown to help people with high blood pressure reduce their levels. Exercise also seems to prevent what used to be

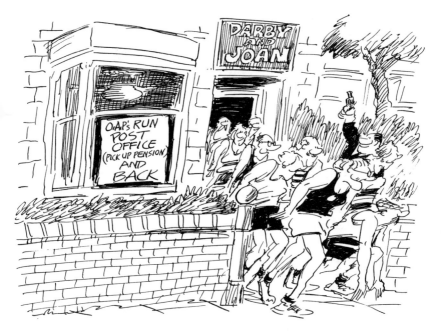

thought of as the inevitable increase in blood pressure as people get older.

Third, a number of studies have suggested that exercise seems to help people give up smoking. It is not clear if people are using exercise as a coping strategy while they are trying to stop, or if people who exercise give up smoking to improve their performance. None the less, one study even showed that, of the smokers who took up running, three-quarters of them stopped smoking.

Exercise also seems to affect coronary heart disease indirectly in a number of ways. For example, although it is perfectly acceptable to lose weight by eating less energy(calorie)-rich food (particularly fat), you can speed up the process of losing weight by exercising. Exercise not only increases the amount of energy (calories) used by the body while you are exercising, it also probably encourages your body to keep on using energy (calories) for a number of hours afterwards. So, if you go for a run before your evening meal, you could still be using up more energy (calories) than normal much later on while you're watching TV!

111

Don't worry about exercise making you hungrier. Exercise doesn't necessarily increase your appetite and some results show that it can even reduce it. What *has* been shown is that people who exercise regularly often eat more food than 'couch potatoes', but don't put on weight because they use up all the extra energy (calories).

Another paradox is that, even though you're speeding up the process of losing weight your scales might be telling you it's happening more slowly. As you exercise, your body is using up fat stores and building up your muscles. But muscle is heavier than fat so if, for example, you've lost two kilos (four pounds) in *weight* you may actually have lost four kilos (eight pounds) of *fat*. Incidentally, muscle can also help to improve your body shape and tone and can also improve your posture, which may help with back problems.

Exercise has been shown to affect another indirect risk factor in coronary heart disease: diabetes. Diabetics who do not have to take insulin injections can use exercise as well as diet as a method of controlling the level of sugar in their blood. Even insulin-dependent diabetics can take exercise, provided they are careful about the timing of their injections and their meals. Some diabetics have gone on to be top class sportsmen and women.

Exercise can also help to reduce stress (see chapter eight). In at least one study exercise proved to be as effective as psychotherapy in treating people with mild depression. Other research has indicated that regular exercise can reduce anxiety, help people to sleep better and generate a feeling of well-being.

Exercising the heart muscle

Finally, exercise exercises the heart muscle too. In many ways the heart muscle is similar to the muscles in the arms and legs and, although the heart muscle is constantly moving, if it isn't given a little extra, regular work to do, it can become 'lazy'. Exercise makes the heart muscle strong enough to pump more blood with each beat and improves the efficiency of the lungs so that more oxygen is obtained from air that is breathed in. This means that when you're resting, the heart can pump more slowly – more blood with each beat and more oxygen from each breath allows your body to get all the oxygen it needs with fewer beats. This, in turn, puts less strain on your heart. A fit heart also has an improved reserve capacity, so that when you're not resting, for example, doing the shopping or digging the garden, your heart can provide the extra oxygen without straining and your stamina improves.

Given this long list of ways in which exercise can reduce your coronary risk – improving blood cholesterol and blood pressure levels, keeping your weight under control, helping you cope with stress and the everyday demands of your life – you would expect that at least some of these benefits would last a few years, even after you'd stopped exercising. The fact that the benefits don't last has led scientists to investigate not only those factors which might help prevent the chronic build up of coronary atherosclerosis but also what might prevent the acute phase of the disease – the heart attack. We shall look at exercise for coronary patients in more detail in chapter nine but preliminary results seem to show that exercise can inhibit some clotting factors in the blood, so reducing the chances of thrombosis and blockage of the coronary arteries. Exercise also seems to reduce the likelihood of problems with the heart's natural rhythm, i.e. the pacemaker difficulties which can complicate coronary heart disease.

All this is bad news for people who have given up the sporting life, but excellent news if you thought it was far too late to bother with exercise as a means of reducing your risk of coronary heart disease.

Many people in the UK clearly think it *is* too late to bother with exercise (or have some other reason why they don't exercise) because participation rates are low and rising only slowly. In 1977 only 35 per cent of men said they had been involved in any outdoor recreational activity in the previous week and this had crept up to 40 per cent some ten years later. Women seem to be even less interested in exercise, with only 21 per cent participating in an outdoor activity in 1977 and a mere 24 per cent ten years on. However, there has been quite a marked increase in the number of women taking up indoor activities such as keep-fit classes and this is an encouraging sign.

None the less, there is plenty of room for improvement. But before you leap up to transform yourself from a couch potato into a runner bean, there are a few important guidelines.

How much exercise should I do?

No matter how keen you are to get fit, start at an easy pace and build up slowly. The more unfit you are and the older you are, the more gradual the approach to exercise should be (but the more you will benefit). Suddenly increasing the amount of exercise will 'surprise' your body, making it much more likely that the muscles will be strained or injured.

Basically, if you begin to feel pain, it is a sign that you have overdone it and you should stop. Going through the pain barrier might be all right for highly trained athletes but it is wrong for anyone else. If the pain, or any other unusual symptom, doesn't go away when you stop or slow down, consult your doctor so you can find out what is causing it.

When to consult your doctor

You should also go and see your doctor *before* you start to exercise if any of the following apply to you:

High blood pressure

You may not know what your blood pressure is because you have never had it checked, or the last time you did was more than five years ago. Your doctor will check it for you. If you do have high blood pressure this does not mean that you can't exercise. In fact, it is more important for you to exercise because the extra activity may help to bring your blood pressure down. You just need to be more careful than someone without high blood pressure. Pay particular attention to the gradual build-up and avoid the kinds of exercise that require power, strength and explosive effort such as press-ups, lifting heavy weights, sit-ups, squash, sprinting and isometric or static exercises such as pushing your hands together as hard as you can. All of these can cause a sharp increase in your blood pressure while performing the exercise.

Chest pains or chest trouble such as asthma or bronchitis

Chapter nine gives more information for people with angina. But with other chest diseases, you have more to gain from being active. The level of exercise you will be able to manage will clearly depend on the severity of your condition, but many people find that swimming is far less likely to make them 'wheezy' than many other activities. And just plain walking is an excellent form of exercise, particularly because you can instantly slow down or stop if you feel a bit under par, or speed up if you're doing well.

Back trouble, or pain in other joints such as arthritis

Swimming is often ideal if you have back or joint problems because you become almost weightless in water and this takes the strain off your joints. The two main problems with swimming are, first, you might never have learned how to swim and second, you might not live near a swimming pool (rivers and the sea are not recommended for swimming because, in the event of your getting into difficulties, there may be no one there to help). There's not much you can do about the second problem but there are plenty of classes to teach you how to swim (and to help you get over a fear of water, if that's the problem) for people of all ages.

Diabetes

Diabetes is no bar to fitness and in fact exercise can help to control blood sugar levels. If you are diabetic, your doctor will provide helpful advice on the timing of food intake and insulin injections (if you need them).

A cold or virus

Viral infections can sometimes affect the heart muscle and if you exercise before you've fully recovered this can make any heart infection worse. It just isn't worth the risk, so wait until your cold, flu or other virus has cleared up.

Recovering from an illness or operation

This is just common sense really, but your doctor or specialist should be able to advise you when it's safe to start exercising – either again or for the first time. The watchword, of course, is gradual.

If you're worried about any other aspect of your health it's always worth checking with your doctor first. GPs are increasingly interested in exercise and can help put your mind at rest, so you can put your body to work.

What kind of exercise and how often?

How often?

In some ways, the more frequent the exercise the better. If you can exercise for just 10 minutes or so every day you'll be surprised at how much fitter you feel. But there's no need to exercise every day: two or three times a week for 20 to 30 minutes will do, and even an hour once a week is better than nothing at all. So long as exercise is regular – and it really *does* need to be every week – the precise timings aren't that crucial. Don't worry if you have to have a break from your exercise routine for some reason. Just start exercising again at a more gentle pace than when you left off and build up again gradually.

Type of exercise

Using oxygen is the critical part of exercising to help prevent coronary heart disease. Aerobic means 'with oxygen' and describes the type of exercise in which the large muscles in your arms, legs and back are regularly expanding and contracting at a steady pace. When the muscles move in this way they need more oxygen, so you breathe more frequently and deeply to take in more oxygen and your heart beats faster to pump the oxygen-rich blood to the muscles more rapidly. A steady, rhythmic movement of the muscles means the heart and lungs can gradually increase their work rate to increase the amount of oxygen in the system and at the same time improve their own efficiency.

There are all kinds of different calculations you can do, depending on your age and your resting and exercising pulse rate, to see if your particular exercise is aerobic or not. A much simpler way is to exercise to the point where you're *slightly* out of breath and you can feel your heart beating a little faster – a pretty good indication that your lungs and heart are working a bit harder. You should still have enough breath to be able to talk (to yourself if you're on your own!) and if you can't – slow down. This type of exercise is also sometimes known as dynamic or isotonic activity and will improve your stamina.

The opposite of aerobic exercise is anaerobic, static or isometric exercise. This is exercise for muscle strength (see page 114). Because the muscles move very quickly then stop again, extra oxygen just can't get there fast enough, hence the term anaerobic – 'without oxygen'. Aerobic exercise to improve your stamina will increase your muscle strength to some degree. Once you're fit, if you want to increase your strength, anaerobic exercises are fine but not at all necessary.

Choosing exercise

There's not much point in putting all this effort into getting fit if you don't keep it up. That's why it's so important that you choose an activity that you enjoy. Better still, choose several activities so that you won't get bored and if the weather or facilities aren't right for one type of exercise you can do one of the others. Best of all is to make exercise so much a part of your daily life that you hardly notice it.

Because the car is such an ingrained part of life in modern Britain people often forget that walking used to be our main method of transport. The human body is very well adapted to walking and as a form of exercise it has a long list of advantages: for example, it's cheap (all you need is a comfortable pair of shoes), and it's flexible – walking pace can be adapted to any level of fitness to work up to your optimal level of fitness. And you can do it practically any time, anywhere.

Cycling is another form of exercise-as-transport and, apart

from the initial expense and a little maintenance, has all the advantages of walking and is a lot quicker. The vigorous cyclists among the British civil servants mentioned before had low coronary heart disease rates: but *any* cycling is a good, aerobic method of exercising and is likely to be above your normal level of activity. There are, of course, some drawbacks to cycling, for example, if you have to travel in a congested town centre.

Once you've walked or cycled to your destination, keep moving. Unless you have heavy weights to carry, walk up the escalators and avoid the lift. Steadily climbing the stairs can add valuable extra minutes to your aerobic total for the week. Go for a walk at lunchtime too.

To add to this (or instead, if daily activity really isn't practical for you) there is a wide range of aerobic activities you can do by yourself and at your own pace. Exercising alone can be a valuable escape from the day's chores or just be a way of getting fitter before you 'go public'. Either way, any of the following might appeal: jogging, running, skipping, swimming, skating. Some need specific facilities or equipment, some don't need much at all. Any of them, of course, could be done with a friend or in a group. Hill-walking is a good group activity.

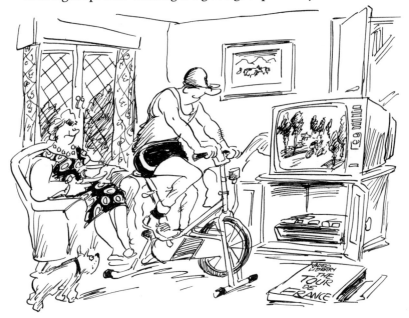

Once you're fitter you may also consider getting an exercise tape or video, or an exercise machine of some type so that you don't need to leave the privacy of your own home. The main problem is that you need to be very motivated indeed to use them regularly. Exercise tapes or machines, because of their repetitive nature, can be very boring. Music can help, of course, or listening to something on headphones at the same time could make it more interesting. A recent report by Consumers' Association on some exercise machines highlights the need to check the safety of the machines before you buy. You should make sure that the machines are stable and comfortable when in use and that they have adjustable features so that they are safe for you to use and meet your individual requirements for exercise, i.e. whether the machine is best for stamina, strength or flexibility training.

Join a class or club

Many people realise that, on their own, they're just not likely to keep going with their exercise programme so they exercise with a friend or with a group of people. Tennis, badminton, table tennis, dancing, aerobics classes and keep-fit are all adaptable to various levels of skill and the intensity can be increased as you improve. Most sports centres run coaching courses suitable for all levels, from beginners to advanced. Squash and team games such as football, netball, hockey and so on are better for keeping fit rather than getting fit because of the temptation to overdo it. At the other end of the scale, quite relaxing sports such as bowls can be helpful if your level of fitness is quite low and you walk around briskly enough. It's not necessary to be a member of a gym to get fit: making use of local facilities such as the park or exercise classes in the church hall will be just as effective.

Are there any risks to activity?

You may have heard of Jim Fixx, the American guru of jogging, who dropped dead while out on his daily run. But you probably don't know that a number of his close family had coronary heart disease, that he also had well-advanced coronary heart disease and that he had been ignoring one of the cardinal rules of exercise – if it hurts, stop. Although exercise probably prolonged his life, it would probably have kept him going even longer if he had listened to his body. Coronary deaths during exercise are rare, which could be the reason why they make the news.

Not only do exercisers have much lower death rates from coronary heart disease, but they also have lower death rates in general. The real danger is *occasional* vigorous exercise. Exercise must be regular – if you've had a break for some reason, start again gradually.

Some people fear that they will spend most of the time injured if they play regular sport. Obviously some sports are more dangerous than others, but if you stick to the guidelines – start gradually, build up slowly and take notice of warning signs – you should be fine. You shouldn't be involved in very strenuous activities anyway unless you are already fit, and even the fittest athlete knows the importance of warming up to avoid any immediate strain on the muscles. It's also sensible (and more comfortable) to exercise before you eat, or wait three or four hours after a meal. When your food is being digested, extra blood is being diverted to the gut, so to ask your heart to provide extra for exercise may be asking for trouble.

Qualifications to look for:

- The Basic Certificate in the Teaching of Exercise to Music is awarded after completion of a course approved by the Royal Society of Arts Examination Board in association with the Sports Council
- Membership of Asset: the National Association for Health and Exercise Teachers
- Teaching certificates awarded by recognised national organisations such as:
  British Slimnastics Association
  Keep Fit Association
  Margaret Morris Movement
  Medau Society and Women's League of Health and Beauty

For further information, contact the Central Council of Physical Recreation on 071-828 3163.

Proper training should also help you avoid injury problems. A qualified teacher (see below) will show you the correct techniques and not encourage you to go beyond your limits. This is where joining a class or a club has an advantage over exercising alone and the social aspect is more enjoyable too.

Being overweight

People who are overweight may feel that exercise is too risky for them. Unless you are very overweight (in which case your doctor will be able to advise you) there is no reason why, if you follow the guidelines, you shouldn't become as fit as anyone else. It might take you a little longer, but you have everything to gain and only your weight to lose.

Age

Others might worry that they're too old to start running around a sports pitch. There are a number of older people who might disagree with that, but in any case, there are plenty of activities which would be enough to get you slightly out of breath. And that's all it takes. In some ways regular exercise is more important the older you are because it not only helps to reduce your risk of coronary heart disease, but if you do the right kind of flexibility exercises it can help you stay more mobile and, therefore, independent. Exercise will also improve your circulation – a boon if you suffer from cold hands and feet. Some sports centres run special exercise programmes for the over-50s. There are exercise evening classes aimed at this age-group too.

Exercise is particularly important for older women because it can help to slow down the process of osteoporosis, or thinning of the bones. Bone is living tissue which can get stronger or weaker, just like muscle. Although bones don't get stronger in the same way as muscle, they respond to the same treatment – exercise. With age there is an inevitable decline in the strength of muscles and bones; in women this begins to accelerate after the menopause. This is why older women so often suffer from broken bones if they fall. Exercise can slow down this weakening process, making the bones less brittle and less likely to fracture.

Finally, what about the other end of the age spectrum – children? Detailed surveys undertaken at Exeter University have shown that children are nowhere near as active as they should be for their health. Television and computer games are gaining ground from cycling or playing in the park and even quite young childen are spending large periods of time doing nothing more strenuous than watching a flickering screen. By far the best solution to this is to get active with your children. Simply telling them to go out and play while *you* watch the television reinforces the idea that exercise is childish. Virtually all of the activities mentioned so far are just as suitable for children and it's important for children to experience a variety of games and sports. It increases the chances of their finding something that they like and reduces the likelihood of their being put off exercise for life. The following 'equation' may help you to remember the advice on exercise:

Frequent + Use oxygen + Now = FUN!

CHAPTER 8

WHAT YOU CAN DO – REDUCE STRESS

SOME researchers believe that stress is a significant risk factor for coronary heart disease. Many people's image of the type of person most likely to have a heart attack is of the over-stressed, frantic and ambitious executive in a high-powered job. But executive types are actually far less likely to suffer from coronary heart disease than their colleagues on the factory floor.

A large part of the difficulty in establishing a link between stress and coronary heart disease, and one of the main reasons why it is such a controversial area even in scientific circles, is that stress is very difficult to define. High-flying executives, for example, might look stressed but they might actually have chosen that type of job because they find it exciting, challenging and enjoyable. Are they more, or less, stressed than an elderly person, living alone, with no friends or relatives nearby and only a pension to get by on? Or the middle-aged person whose marriage has just ended in divorce and the loss of the family home?

All of these people might be under tremendous stress. But the pensioner might be finding retirement a wonderful period of relaxation and fulfilment after years of grinding employment, and divorce might be a joyful release from a traumatic relationship. It is therefore difficult to define stress simply by looking at a person's situation.

There have been many attempts to define stress and one of the most famous theories was developed by Mayer Friedman and Ray Rosenman in America in the 1950s. They classified people as two basic types: Type A individuals, who are aggressive, impatient, competitive, always in a rush, never satisfied and generally workaholics; and Type B individuals, who are calm, easy-going and patient. Their research showed that Type A individuals are more likely to suffer from coronary heart disease than Type Bs.

Results from the Framingham study supported this idea (see page 184). Type A people in the town did indeed seem to suffer higher rates of coronary heart disease. The stress factor seemed to be particularly relevant for Type As who were men in white-collar jobs. This is not so surprising because Mayer Friedman and Ray Rosenman developed the theory by studying people who, by and large, *were* men in white-collar jobs. Others might have been predicted that the theory would not hold for different groups of people.

In fact, one of the largest studies, MRFIT (see page 184), could find no link at all between Type A people and coronary heart disease. More doubt was cast on the theory when a ten-year study of 18,000 civil servants in London found that it seemed to work in reverse! Type A behaviour was more common in the higher grades of the civil service but coronary heart disease rates were highest in the lowest grades – three times higher.

The difference between the grades couldn't be entirely explained by the main risk factors – blood cholesterol, blood pressure and smoking – but the 'personality' theory of stress didn't seem to explain it either. Yet researchers didn't abandon the idea of stress, they tried to find another, broader theory which would include the stressful events which happened to someone, as well as the way the person reacts to them – the social causes of stress as well as the psychological reaction – the psychosocial approach to linking stress and coronary heart disease.

Psychosocial stress

A good deal of evidence has accumulated to support this theory. Bereavement, for example, is a very stressful event and coronary rates have been found to be higher among the recently bereaved. Unemployment too can place a huge burden on individuals and families and the Scottish Heart Health Study and others found higher coronary rates in areas of high unemployment than elsewhere. But even having a job can be a mixed blessing and research from Sweden showed that where people had little control over the kind of work they did or the pace of it – for example on a production line – coronary heart disease rates were higher than expected.

Employment is not the only aspect of 'psychosocial' stress. Studies of people who have emigrated have shown increased coronary rates. The problem seems most acute in a particular generation of immigrants. The parents seem to cope quite well with their new life. This is much as you would expect, since they have made the difficult choice to leave their homes and are strongly motivated to succeed in their new life. Their grand-children, too, seem to suffer little stress, since they are usually born in the new country and know no other way of life. But the middle generation often have roots in both societies and the stress of feeling torn between two cultures may lead to increased rates of coronary heart disease.

A similar phenomenon has been observed in people who move from rural areas to town and cities, but other research has shown that it is possible to avoid some of the stress of migration. Michael Marmot's study of Japanese families who moved to America showed that those who maintained the intricate networks of family support fared much better than the Japanese families who adopted the less structured American way of life. The notion of family support relieving stress has also been shown in other research where, for example, people who have never married also have higher rates of coronary heart disease (though this seems to apply to men who do not marry and not to women who stay single).

Stress in women

As more women move into paid employment outside the home and also, because of equal opportunities, take on jobs which used to be thought of as 'men's work', some commentators have suggested that women will begin to suffer more from stress and increase their rates of 'male' diseases, particularly coronary heart disease. There are two flaws to this argument: first, coronary heart disease never has been simply a man's disease. Women suffer almost as much angina as men and, after the menopause, have almost the same risk of dying of a heart attack as men.

Second, current research from the Framingham study shows that women in well-paid, satisfying jobs do not suffer higher rates of coronary heart disease. This is borne out by statistics in the USA which show falling coronary rates among both women and men while female employment rates have been steadily rising. What Framingham did show, however, was that women in low paid, low status, boring jobs had higher coronary rates than their more fortunate colleagues in better paid, more interesting jobs.

So although it is difficult to pinpoint exactly what we mean by stress, there is a good deal of evidence to show that some combination of the stressful events that happen to us, and the way we react to them, has some bearing on whether or not we develop coronary heart disease. And there are convincing explanations as to how stress might damage the coronary arteries.

The stress response

When you are faced with a stressful event there is a series of predictable reactions in the body. Hormones, such as adrenalin, are immediately released into the system. You begin to breathe more quickly and your heart rate shoots up. Your body is trying to get as much oxygen and nutrients as possible to the muscles and the brain to prepare to 'fight' the danger, or run away from it – 'flight'. Blood supply is redirected away from the skin and the digestion to let even more blood get to the muscles, and the heart helps by beating faster and increasing the pressure in the system. Extra fats, such as cholesterol, and sugar are released into the bloodstream, so the muscles have an instant supply of energy (calories). The body prepares for the possibility of injury by releasing other substances into the blood to make it more likely to clot and so heal wounds faster.

If the source of your stress was a sabre-toothed tiger this

would all be extremely useful: you probably wouldn't choose to grapple with it, but your body would be ready to make a speedy exit! The body's stress response is less useful if you have just watched a party political broadcast by your least favourite politician. The human body still reacts in a primitive way to stress, in a wide variety of situations. The blood pressure rises (increasing the likelihood of damage to the delicate artery lining), the cholesterol in our blood is not used up (so might build up on the artery walls) and the blood is still sticky (and might form a clot to block an artery).

Stress can also affect coronary heart disease indirectly. Many smokers smoke more cigarettes in the mistaken belief that it helps them to relax. Another common response to stress, with an indirect effect on general health, is to reach for the biscuit tin, or go to the sweet shop, or take comfort in some other type of food. People rarely reach for a carrot when they're feeling angry or depressed and sweet and fatty foods can pile up the calories and put on the pounds, with the resultant health risk that being overweight entails.

Even riskier is a resort to alcohol to dull the pain of stress. The dangers of drinking increasing amount of alcohol go far beyond that of putting on weight.

Dealing with stress

Dealing with stress is a bit like pulling yourself up by your bootstraps, or trying to lift yourself off the ground using your shoelaces – a neat trick and if you knew how to do it you'd have done it before! No one likes feeling stressed and everyone would deal with it if they could. But when you're right in the thick of it, dealing with stress seems just as impossible as defying the laws of gravity.

Sometimes stress isn't just a result of one event or even several events all happening at the same time. The stress you feel may be related to your family, your work, your home – in other words, part of your life. So asking someone to deal with stress is like asking them to change their life – in some cases, an impossible request.

None of the suggestions below for dealing with stress is

going to change your life. Just as with giving up smoking or changing your diet, there are no miraculous short-cuts. No matter how hopeless your particular stressful situation might seem there is nearly always something, no matter how small, that can be done to improve it. Some of the techniques we describe may be all you need. Some people will need more specialist help and even knowing that there is professional help may be a relief.

Dealing with stress can be approached in two ways: coping with its effects and dealing with its causes. Most stress-relieving techniques concentrate on helping individuals to find ways of coping. This is like trying to cure measles by putting calamine lotion on the spots – it makes measles more bearable but does nothing to prevent or cure the disease. But there's no denying that soothing the 'itchy spots' of stress can be useful.

Coping with stress

There are three main ways of coping with the effects of stress and reducing the damage that the stress response, the 'fight or flight' mechanism, may be doing to your heart: breathing exercises, muscle relaxation and meditation.

Relaxation
Learning how to breathe may seem a little bizarre considering you do it automatically between 16,000 and 20,000 times a day. But deep, relaxed and steady breathing is completely different to the rapid, shallow breaths you take when you're feeling stressed.

Breathing for relaxation
Place your right hand, lightly, on your stomach with your left hand resting on your chest. Keep your mouth closed and breathe slowly through your nose. As you breathe out, pull your stomach muscles in and then let them relax as you breathe in. Your left hand should stay still, while your right hand will move as the air flows in and out of your lungs. After a few breaths, relax your stomach muscles and let them move in and out naturally. Don't force yourself to breathe extra slowly or

more deeply than usual, just concentrate on breathing gently through your nose, with your left hand staying still on your chest and your right, rising and falling with each breath.

Take five minutes, each day, to practise this breathing technique. Some people prefer to do this exercise lying down (a good reason for not eating beforehand) but sitting down or standing up will do just as well. This type of breathing – abdominal or diaphragmatic breathing – helps to fill the lungs with oxygen and get rid of the excess carbon dioxide. Shallow breathing tends to take in less oxygen and leave some carbon dioxide in the lungs. In fact you could try the breathing exercise next time you feel stressed (if circumstances allow it) and see if it helps to calm you down.

Muscle relaxation
Muscle relaxation is the next stage on from this gentle breathing. Again, some people prefer to lie on the floor, but you can do it sitting at your desk, for example, or while a passenger in a car. So long as it's somewhere reasonably comfortable and warm, anywhere will do.

First of all you need to get a slow, steady breathing rhythm going (after some practice you'll probably be able to do it without putting your hands on your chest and stomach). Once you're breathing softly and feeling quite relaxed, close your eyes and concentrate on your feet. Imagine they feel warm and heavy and every single toe and all the muscles are completely loose and relaxed. Then focus on your calf muscles, your knees, your thighs, your hands, your back, and so on, all the way up to your face – taking all the time you need to let the tension float out of each group of muscles, leaving them totally relaxed. Keep that warm, relaxed feeling for a few moments, concentrating on the steady rhythm of your breathing. When you're ready, wriggle your fingers and toes a little, take a deep breath and open your eyes. Then take a good stretch.

A common variant of this technique is to tense each group of muscles first before you relax them. This emphasises the contrast between tense and relaxed muscles. Some people find it easier to do the exercise this way, at least at first, until they get used to the 'feel' of their muscles. This is fine if it suits you better but it's not necessary and, if you have high blood pressure, the tensing action might cause a slight, temporary increase in your blood pressure.

Meditation
Breathing exercises alone, or combined with muscle relaxation, may be enough to help you cope with the smaller stresses and strains of daily life, but some people will benefit from meditation. Meditation requires a very quiet, private place and far more perseverance. But many find it well worth the effort. Meditation includes breathing exercises and muscle relaxation but goes on to focus the mind on a single object or word, to the exclusion of every other thought.

The popularity, and hence presumably effectiveness, of these relaxation techniques either singly or in combination, has led to an explosion of books, tapes, videos and classes on relaxation as a method of coping with stress. There are no formal qualifications for teachers of relaxation techniques, but some of the associations listed at the back of the book should be able to provide more details. There are also variations on the relaxation theme, such as the Alexander Technique, yoga, biofeedback and autogenics (see page 187 for their central office addresses).

There is no harm in trying any of these exercises. At the very least, you won't be doing, or thinking about, whatever it is that makes you feel stressed. There is also evidence to show that people with high blood pressure who take to relaxation techniques can reduce their blood pressure levels, not only during the exercise, but permanently.

Talking
'A problem shared is a problem halved' is one of the oldest clichés, but, like most such phrases, it has become over-used because it has a grain of truth. A good place to start talking over a problem is with yourself! If, for example, you are standing at the bus stop, it's pouring down with rain and you are late, it is likely that you feel stressed. You're wet, miserable and worried that your friends will think you are not coming and leave without you. Ask yourself if it is really worth getting wound up about. So you're wet: it's only water and it will dry. Is it your

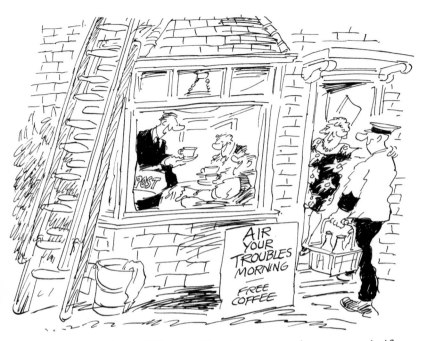

fault the bus is late? Will your friends never speak to you again if you're late? It is hardly likely. Maybe you could go home early instead and watch that repeat of your favourite sitcom?

Of course not all stressful situations can be dealt with in this way, but some of life's little niggles, which can often build up into a major cause of stress, can, if looked at in a different way, become much less of a strain.

Talking to someone else can be a boon. If your problem is leading you in vicious circles, a friend can sometimes spot how to break that circle and at least start the process of trying to solve the problem. Even if the friend or relative cannot offer much practical help, just being there and listening can help lift the burden from your shoulders. This might be how family support systems helped the Japanese immigrants cope with their new lives in the United States. Further evidence for the 'being there' theory comes from studies which show that single people who have had heart attacks live longer if they have a pet than those who don't. It may be the affection that pets show their owners, or just physical contact with another living creature that seems to work.

If you feel that your family or friends *are* the problem, there are a range of 'professional listeners' who might be able to help. Marriage guidance counsellors are trained to deal with a wide range of family problems and unmarried couples can also take advantage of their services. Your doctor may be happy to refer you to any one of a range of specialists that might include psychiatrists, psychologists, psychotherapists and psychoanalysts. There is also a range of alternative counselling techniques (see page 130).

Exercise

In addition to, or instead of, any of the above ways of coping with stress, you could try reacting in an active way. If your body is all geared up for action then why not exercise? The best time to do it, of course, is at the moment you feel stressed but your colleagues may not appreciate you leaving, in the middle of a difficult meeting, to pop out for a run round the park. With a little imagination, though, a brisk walk round the block or steadily climbing a few flights of stairs for five minutes can be worked into most situations. An alternative option is to take time later in the day, or later in the week, to run, cycle, swim or any of the other aerobic activities described in chapter seven. As well as helping to reduce stress exercising will bring a whole range of other benefits for your health.

Assertiveness

Assertiveness as a way of dealing with stress sits at a kind of halfway point between coping with stress and tackling the causes. Assertiveness is not to be confused with being aggressive. Aggressive behaviour is that in which people act as if their needs are the most important in the world. The opposite of aggressive behaviour is passive behaviour. The passive child, for example, is often mercilessly teased at school.

These are stereotypes of course. Hardly anyone is aggressive or passive all the time, but on balance, their behaviour falls into one camp or the other. This is similar to the 'Type A and Type B' theory of stress (see page 123) but with a number of differences. Learning to be assertive is learning how to change your behaviour rather than your whole personality. Assertiveness training also tends to focus as much, if not more, on people who are passive – the type Bs. Quiet types may not show their stress as much as the aggressive type, but it does not mean that they never feel it. Hiding your emotions can be just as damaging to your heart as storming about the place slamming doors.

Like meditation, learning to be assertive is not something which can be picked up from a few paragraphs in a book. Complete training courses and publications about assertiveness are available but the following may give you something of the flavour of the approach. The core of assertiveness 'training' is to learn to value yourself. Much of the training on assertiveness courses centres around practising how to be assertive in mockups of real situations, such as taking shoddy goods back to a shop and learning how to say 'no thank you' to another piece of Auntie Flo's chocolate cake without caving in.

These are trivial examples and at root, becoming assertive is another 'bootstrapping' operation. But, with practice, people have found that assertiveness training has given them the resilience to cope with some of the stresses in their lives and sometimes even the confidence to tackle the causes of their problems.

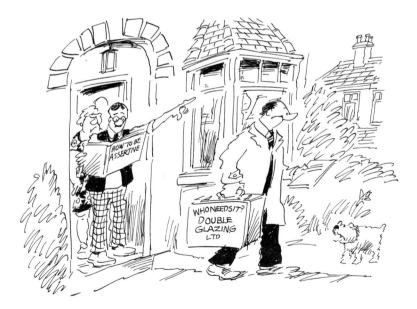

Dealing with the causes of stress

Having hoisted yourself up by your bootstraps you could begin to tackle the cause of your stress. Step number one is to break the problem or problems up into smaller and potentially more manageable pieces. If you say your problem is 'work', set out *exactly* what is it about work that is causing you stress: the pay, the physical conditions (too noisy, crowded, dangerous), a particular person or people, a certain situation, the travelling involved?

Take each part in turn and work out what could be done to make the situation better. For example, you could discuss your problem with a sympathetic member of staff, inform the health and safety officer about the unsafe conditions, talk to the person who is driving you mad (he or she might not realise the effect that he or she is having) and try to work out an alternative method of getting to work. Not all of the problems need be tackled by you alone. If there is a union or staff association, perhaps it could step up negotiations with the management for improved pay and conditions. The personnel officer might be able to act as intermediary in inter-departmental squabbles.

Perhaps there are external experts you could turn to. If the problem is not just low pay, for example, but you're also faced with an unexpectedly high bill, you might need financial advice. Banks, building societies and the customer services departments of the gas, electricity and telephone companies will be able to give you advice. Try a Citizens Advice Bureau (or Debt Counselling Service) who will have information on how to defer payments, or on benefits to which you may be entitled.

There is no guarantee that this approach will wipe away all sources of stress in your life but it is important to realise that there are people out there who can help. You don't even need to turn to professional experts if you don't want to, or perhaps can't afford to. There are usually hundreds, perhaps thousands, of people who are in a similar situation or who have been through it and lived to tell the tale. They too are experts. There are thousands of voluntary organisations, self-help groups, charities, action committees and community associations all over the country that may be of help to you. It is more than likely that at least one of them specialises in a problem which affects you.

Even if these groups have not successfully changed the world yet, they may help you to cope in the meantime.

Like stopping smoking, eating a healthy diet and taking regular exercise, coping with or tackling stress is a fairly low risk strategy for reducing your risk of coronary heart disease. There is no need to fear losing your drive or ambition. Assertive people can achieve just as much, if not more, through quiet determination and planning.

CHAPTER 9

IS IT TOO LATE TO REDUCE YOUR RISK?

UNDERSTANDABLY, many people do not think about coronary heart disease until it affects them personally. You may have bought this book because someone close to you has had a heart attack, or heart surgery, or suffers from angina. You may be reading this book because you already have coronary heart disease. If so, the question, 'Is it too late for you to reduce your risk?' becomes relevant.

There was a time when the answer would have been 'yes'. These days the reply is a resounding 'no!' This chapter will look at secondary prevention, in particular the activities which can improve quality of life and reduce the risk of a second or subsequent attack.

Drugs

A wide range of drugs may be used to deal with coronary heart disease. This section lists the main types of drugs used to treat the disease. This will give you an idea of what to expect if you come across them, or serve as a reminder about what your drugs do, if you are already taking them. It is no substitute, though, for a thorough discussion with your doctor about any drugs he or she might prescribe for your condition. You should certainly know the answers to the following questions.

What is it?

Drugs are often grouped according to what they do (see, for example vasodilators on page 140). A drug will also have an official, or generic name, plus a trade (or proprietary, or brand) name. The proprietary drugs often combine generic drugs in different ways – perhaps one will cancel out the side-effects of the other or make it work more effectively. Drugs also come in different strengths. It is important to remember that, just as people react to the same diet in different ways, people react to the same drug differently. Your doctor may try different drugs or different combinations to find the precise mix which will suit you.

What does it do?

Your doctor should explain what the drug is for and how it will help your particular problem. In some cases it will be obvious. The drug is for pain relief and when you take it the pain goes away. But other drugs, for example those used to reduce blood pressure or blood cholesterol levels, probably won't make you feel any better and might even make you feel worse. If you haven't had any symptoms, and the drug has side-effects, you may wonder why on earth you have to take it. Knowing how the drug is helping, and having regular check-ups to make sure that it is working, will help you persevere with the course of drugs.

What is the dose?

You need to be absolutely clear how many tablets you need to take and how often you need to take them. Some can be taken whenever you need them, while others must be taken at regular intervals. It can be tempting to stop taking a drug if you feel well (or if the side-effects become very unpleasant), but with some drugs, stopping suddenly can be dangerous. You should go back to your doctor and discuss why you want to stop taking the drug. Your doctor may well agree, but don't act without advice.

Are there any side-effects?

Some people experience no problems with drugs, but other people can suffer side-effects that range from mildly unpleasant to positively dangerous. Your doctor should warn you of any possible side-effects so that you are not unduly worried if they develop and you will then be prepared to deal with them. It may mean, for example, that you should not drive, because the drugs make you dizzy. However, you do not have to put up with unpleasant side-effects. There are usually alternative drugs or combinations of drugs which will do the same job but with fewer or possibly no side-effects.

What should you avoid?

The general rule of thumb is that you should avoid alcohol and other drugs: they may interfere with the drug(s) that your doctor has prescribed, making them less effective or producing their own cocktail of side-effects. This doesn't necessarily mean that you have to become teetotal, or not take an aspirin if you have a headache. On the other hand, it might, so ask.

If you think you might get flustered or forget to ask any of these questions, write them down – and the answers that you get. Your doctor will be pleased to give you the information because a well-informed patient who understands the treatment

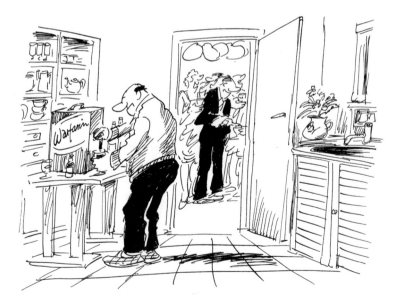

is more likely to stick to it and to report any changes in symptoms which might be important.

Vasodilators

The vasodilators are a group of drugs which, in various ways, dilate the blood vessels, both the arteries and veins, making it much easier for blood to flow through them. These drugs are often used for people with high blood pressure or angina.

Nitrates

Nitrates have been used for very many years to help relieve the pain of angina. They are based on nitro-glycerine (an ingredient used in dynamite). There are fast-acting nitrates which can be used for the immediate relief of an angina attack. These need to be absorbed into the bloodstream quickly so they are placed near the surface of the body, where there is a rich supply of blood vessels, for example under the tongue. A nasal spray has also been developed. Slower-acting nitrates can also be taken regularly to prevent angina attacks.

The problem with nitrates is that they relax all the arteries and veins, not just the coronary arteries, so that when you first start to take them, you may get a flushing sensation or headaches. These effects usually wear off once you have got used to the drug.

Calcium antagonists

These drugs relax the blood vessels by 'mopping up' the calcium in the artery walls and making them less tough. This is particularly useful if spasm (the sudden narrowing of the arteries) is a problem, because calcium antagonists make the contractions much weaker. Fluid retention and dizziness are two possible side-effects.

ACE-inhibitors

These are a newer type of vasodilator: they work by inhibiting or interfering with the angiotensin-converting enzyme or ACE. Angiotensin is one of the chemicals in the body responsible for narrowing the blood vessels. By reducing this enzyme's ability to narrow the blood vessels, the ACE-inhibitors keep the blood vessels relaxed. Unlike calcium antagonists, the ACE-inhibitors may encourage the body to lose too much fluid and they may also upset the functioning of the kidneys.

Diuretics

Diuretic drugs have been used for a long time to help lower blood pressure. They are often known as water tablets because they work by encouraging the body to lose water and salt. Some diuretics also help the body to conserve potassium at the same time. By altering the balance of minerals and reducing the volume of fluid, these drugs can be quite effective in reducing blood pressure. Unfortunately they are not suitable for diabetics and may, like ACE-inhibitors, lead to excess loss of fluid, leaving you feeling weak and a little dizzy. Some men taking diuretics find that they cannot maintain an erection. If this happens, you should certainly talk to your doctor, who can put you onto another drug.

Beta-blockers

Beta-blockers are useful for angina sufferers and for preventing another heart attack. This group of drugs works by blocking the activity of the stress hormones, for example adrenalin, and so reduces both the strength of the heart beat and the number of beats per minute. A slower, weaker heart beat means the heart needs much less oxygen, so the beta-blockers can reduce the strain on the furred up arteries which are trying to supply the oxygen-rich blood. Unfortunately one of the other functions of adrenalin is to keep the body's breathing tubes open, so if you interfere with adrenalin, these airways tend to constrict. This makes beta-blockers unsuitable for people with asthma, bronchitis or other breathing disorders. Beta-blockers also tend to make the peripheral vessels narrow, so if you have peripheral vessel disease (see page 32 in chapter two) you would not be prescribed these drugs. Even for people without this problem, beta-blockers can cause cold hands and feet. They also have a tendency to make people feel tired or suffer from nightmares.

Digoxin

One of the oldest known heart drugs also changes the heart rate. Digoxin – from the foxglove (or digitalis) – slows the heart down but, unlike beta-blockers, increases the force of the beats. This is particularly useful if, due to coronary heart disease or another cause, your heart muscle is not pumping properly and heart failure has developed.

Blood-thinning drugs

Anticoagulants
Anticoagulants are often used to try to thin the blood. By far the most common drug for this purpose is warfarin, also known as rat poison. The dosage for this drug has to be set very carefully. If it is too low, it doesn't work. If it is too high the blood becomes far too thin. If you are prescribed this drug you will have several blood tests so that the dose can be fine-tuned.

Fish oil capsules
Fish oil capsules may also be used to try to thin the blood, particularly if you have been found to have high levels of triglyceride in your blood. The role of triglycerides in the development of coronary heart disease is not clear, but too high a level of triglycerides in the blood is associated with clotting problems. Fish oil capsules, used with the guidance of a doctor, have been shown to be effective in reducing triglyceride levels.

Antithrombotic drugs
Antithrombotic drugs are used to prevent another problem linked to the stickiness of the blood – a clot or thrombus forming and blocking an artery. Low doses of aspirin have been discovered to be a cheap and effective antithrombotic. However, this does not mean that healthy people should start taking aspirin every day in the hope of preventing a coronary. Although it is a familiar household medicine, aspirin is still a drug and can cause gastro-intestinal problems such as ulcers and internal bleeding. People with coronary heart disease should not simply add aspirin to the drugs the doctor has already

prescribed. This could cause problems: the combination of warfarin and aspirin is particularly dangerous.

If a clot has already formed it may be possible to dissolve it with drugs called thrombolytics, known as 'clot-busters'. One of the most common clot-busters is streptokinase, which is proving particularly valuable in the first few hours after a heart attack. Dissolving the clot which caused the attack can help to get the blood flowing through the coronary arteries again and possibly reduce the damage to the heart muscle.

Cholesterol-lowering drugs

The final group of drugs is used to lower the amount of cholesterol in the blood and, as befits the most studied risk factor for coronary heart disease, there are many different kinds of cholesterol-lowering drugs. Indeed, research is so intense that new types of drugs in this field are being developed all the time. The following are some of the most recent drugs.

Ion-exchange resins
These have been the most common type of drug to deal with blood cholesterol levels. The drugs work by binding themselves with bile-acids in the gut. The body responds to the drop in the level of bile-acids by using cholesterol to make more of these digestive juices. By using up cholesterol, the levels in the bloodstream fall. Unfortunately these drugs, which come as packets of granules, have to be mixed with liquid and taken in large quantities. They can make people feel bloated and sick.

Fibrates
It is not clear how the fibrate drugs reduce cholesterol levels and there is some concern in the medical profession about their long-term safety. Some studies have shown that although deaths from coronary heart disease fall when people take these drugs, deaths from other causes rise. The reasons for this are not clear and this has led the Government's Committee on the Safety of Medicines to be cautious about use of fibrate drugs.

Niacin

Despite the fact that this is a B vitamin, the amount needed to reduce cholesterol levels means it should be treated as a drug. As we noted in chapter six you need to take ten times the recommended daily amount, or more, of niacin and there may be side-effects such as a flushed feeling or liver damage at these levels. The drug is also sometimes known as nicotinic acid and it is more commonly prescribed by doctors in the United States than in Britain.

Fish oil

Although your doctor may prescribe fish oil capsules to help reduce triglyceride levels, it is less likely that they will be prescribed to lower cholesterol levels. Studies have not shown that fish oil capsules are useful in reducing this type of blood fat and more research needs to be done into what the long-term effects of fish oil capsule consumption might be.

Statins

The statins are the latest cholesterol-lowering drug to come on the market. They are based on the Nobel Prize-winning work of Joseph Goldstein and Michael Brown, who discovered that the liver needs 'receptors' to deal with cholesterol and that a genetic defect (FH) and saturated fat interfere with these receptors. Goldstein and Brown also spotted a chemical or enzyme that the body needs to make cholesterol. If this enzyme – HMG. CoA reductase – can be made less effective, it follows that the body will make less cholesterol. The statins are designed to inhibit the workings of this enzyme.

The early results from the testing of these drugs look promising, but long-term studies will be needed to make sure that they don't create the same problems as the fibrates (see page 143) and increase deaths from some other cause.

None of the drugs already described can cure coronary heart disease. They can help ease the pain (the effect of nitrates) or reduce one or more of the risk factors (the use of diuretics for blood pressure or the cholesterol-lowering drugs), or help the heart to cope (the use of beta-blockers). But drugs cannot make coronary heart disease go away and, as we have seen, many of them can have unpleasant side-effects.

Changing your habits

Drugs also should not be used as a substitute for changing your habits. Stopping smoking, changing your diet, taking up exercise and dealing with stress are important for someone with coronary heart disease. For some people, changing their habits might not reduce their risk by a large enough margin for it to be a worthwhile change alone. Your doctor might suggest drugs as well as life-style changes. Even then, the changes you have made can help to reduce the amount of drugs you need. In time, the alterations you have made to your life might enable your doctor to reduce the dose of drugs or even take you off them altogether.

The balance between changing what you do and taking drugs will vary from person to person, depending of course on how severe your coronary problem is and how easily your body reacts to the changes you make. For some people, though, their coronary arteries are in such a state that surgery becomes necessary.

Surgical techniques

Angioplasty

The technique of angioplasty is almost identical to the cardiac catheterisation and angiography procedure described in chapter four (see page 66). A thin plastic tube is inserted into the body via an artery in the arm or leg and guided towards the heart. But, instead of simply examining the coronary arteries, the tube is used to widen the arteries which have become narrowed by atheroma. A balloon is attached to the tube and, when it has been placed at the exact location of the narrowest part of the artery, it is carefully inflated so that the atheroma becomes squashed and the artery is widened.

This technique was developed as recently as 1977 and, although it sounds very simple, like all surgical operations it is never undertaken lightly. You will be under local anaesthetic and will have to stay in hospital for two or three days. Not every case of coronary heart disease is suitable for this kind of treatment and even now it is not really clear how it works. Even when the balloon has been inflated, it is still no wider than three millimetres and researchers are not sure if the balloon pushes the atheroma through the artery wall onto the other side, or stretches the artery, making the whole artery, atheroma and all, wider. Angioplasty does not work if the atheroma is very hard. In about 20 to 30 per cent of cases the artery narrows again, either by a blood clot forming, or by the artery rapidly furring up.

If this happens the procedure can be repeated but, as with angiography, there is always a small risk of the technique triggering a heart attack. The cardiologist may even decide, during the angioplasty, that it would actually be better for you to have a different kind of operation and, rather then bring you back to hospital again, the second operation is performed there and then. About 3 to 4 per cent of angioplasty patients will be transferred in this way, so you will be asked to sign a consent form before your operation in case this happens.

Coronary artery bypass graft

The operation the surgeons will perform is the coronary artery bypass graft (or CABG), sometimes known as 'cabbage'! The surgeon takes a 'spare' bit of healthy blood vessel from somewhere else in your body, cuts it into lengths, attaches one end to the main artery – the aorta – and the other end to a coronary artery, further down from the narrowed or blocked section, thus bypassing the blockage and allowing the blood to flow freely again to that part of the heart muscle. This operation is normally done only if several of the coronary arteries are severely narrowed or blocked, so that you will often hear the operation described as a double or triple coronary bypass operation depending on how many new sections the surgeon sews on.

The first CABG was done in the United States in 1967 and the spare blood vessel was a vein taken from the patient's leg. It is still very common to use a leg vein, but increasingly, cardiac surgeons are using an artery that runs down the inside of the chest wall – the internal mammary artery. This artery seems to fur up less quickly than the leg vein so the chances of a successful operation are increased.

In fact, about 90 per cent of CABGs are successful and the 'new' coronary arteries can remain free of atheroma for years. Not all coronary patients are suitable for CABG: your doctor will have to balance the undoubted benefits against the not inconsiderable risks of a major operation. To be able to operate on your heart the surgeon will split your breastbone and you will be connected to a heart-lung bypass machine which will circulate your blood and breathe for you while the new arteries are being attached. You will be under intensive care for the first two to five days and stay an additional five to ten days in a general ward in the hospital to make sure that no complications develop.

Heart transplant

Perhaps the most famous and dramatic type of heart operation is the heart transplant. Only a few hundred of these operations are performed every year and it is the last resort if the heart's pumping chambers have more or less given up, i.e. if you have severe heart failure. This may be the result of several heart attacks which have left the heart muscle too damaged to be able to pump properly. But heart failure has other causes (see chapter two) so by no means all heart transplant patients have coronary heart disease.

Although around three-quarters of patients survive for a year after this operation and some two-thirds live for five years or more, the operation places an enormous burden on the body so it is usally undertaken only on younger patients. This is a very specialised area of medicine so the guidelines on the secondary prevention of coronary heart disease really are not sufficient for heart transplant patients. Although the guidelines will include the same advice on smoking, diet and exercise, for example, this select band of people will receive additional detailed advice on their recovery.

Secondary prevention

In the past, angina and heart attack sufferers used to have to avoid a long list of activities and face up to long periods of sitting or lying down. The angina would probably get worse, and would be followed by one or more heart attacks and after a little while, death. Even the resting would cause problems. Muscles would weaken and begin to waste away from lack of use and bones would start to get thinner and weaker. The whole body system would become sluggish and constipation might develop. Worse still, blood circulation would be slower, encouraging blood clots to form in the veins, known as deep vein thrombosis. Very often these clots would form in the legs, causing pain and swelling. Sometimes bits of the clot would break off and the resulting embolism could get stuck somewhere else, perhaps in the lungs, causing even more complications in an already serious condition.

Bed rest

It was mainly to avoid these problems of long term bed-rest that some doctors started to encourage their patients to move around a bit more. Sure enough, they had fewer circulation and clotting problems. Problems of increased angina or more heart attacks from the increased workload on the heart did not live up to the doctors' fears. At the same time evidence about the possibilities for preventing coronary heart disease was beginning to build up from studies on smoking, diet, exercise and stress.

Stopping smoking

It is now widely accepted that the single most important action that anyone with coronary heart disease can take is to stop smoking. Studies have shown conclusively that stopping smoking can halve the risk of a second or subsequent heart attack. The pain of angina or the shock of a heart attack is very often all the motivation anyone needs to stop smoking. Stopping smoking will not cure you of heart disease, but it will help to stop your condition getting worse. If your doctor has recommended surgery for you, you should stop smoking before the operation because it will reduce the risk of complications. Some cardiac surgeons refuse to operate on smokers.

Stopping smoking is more effective than taking drugs. Even the most effective drugs developed so far – low doses of aspirin and the beta-blockers – have been shown to reduce coronary deaths by around 25 per cent, compared to 50 per cent for stopping smoking. Drugs to lower blood pressure have failed to demonstrate even a modest effect on coronary death rates (although they have been shown to be important in reducing strokes).

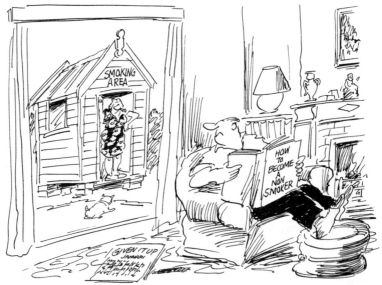

Exercise

Exercise is also at least as effective as some drugs at reducing deaths from coronary heart disease. Although no single study has been able to show an important effect of exercise for people with coronary heart disease, when all the studies are combined, exercise seems to reduce death rates by around 20 per cent. Just as important have been those reports which describe the effects of exercise on the quality of life. People who had previously been crippled with angina or who lived in fear of another heart attack have been able to return to a normal life – in some cases feeling even healthier than before.

Dietary changes

There have been few studies of the effect of dietary changes on the prospects for coronary sufferers. There are clear benefits to losing weight if you are going to have an operation. As with stopping smoking, losing weight reduces the chances of complications after surgery. There is no reason to suppose that the benefits of changing your diet will be any less important for people with coronary heart disease. Some recent research points to a reversal of the process of atherosclerosis in people who adopt a strict low fat diet.

Coping with stress

Although there are problems in defining and studying the relationship between stress and coronary heart disease, research has revealed that some relaxation techniques have allowed doctors to reduce their patients' drug dosage – particularly for blood pressure lowering drugs – and in some cases patients have come off drugs altogether.

Virtually all secondary prevention programmes combine exercise sessions with advice and counselling on stopping smoking, changing diet and learning how to relax. Added to this will be practical help and information on matters which will be of specific interest to people who have had a heart attack or heart surgery or who suffer from angina.

Coping with the emotional ups and downs

A heart attack can be an earth-shattering event for the sufferer, and, unless it has been preceded by angina, will be a terrible shock. Heart attack victims may, not surprisingly, become deeply depressed immediately after the event. They have not yet had to time to come to terms with the fact that they have coronary heart disease and may know very little about the disease. Worst of all, they may believe they will become 'cardiac cripples'. The first few weeks after a heart attack will be a critical time to offer information and, where necessary, psychological support.

In contrast, someone having heart surgery may have a much more positive attitude. They are much more likely to know about their condition and surgery, if successful, holds out the prospect of freedom from pain and the possibility of getting back to 'normal'. But here, too, if surgery is not as successful as hoped, the disappointment can be crushing. Heart surgery is not a magic cure for coronary heart disease and those people who have made 'miraculous' recoveries have done so, not only because of a successful operation, but because they have also changed the way they live their lives.

The problem for angina sufferers is that they may not be offered much in the way of advice on prevention. A heart attack or heart surgery is a major event which can mark the point in your life when you finally decide to *do* something. The gradual development of angina doesn't really present that kind of opportunity and sufferers may gradually become resigned to a lifetime of being on drugs, with little prospect for an improvement in their condition. In fact, angina sufferers have as much to gain from secondary prevention as people on the hospital wards.

What to expect – a typical secondary prevention programme

If you have had a heart attack or heart surgery your doctor will give you detailed advice on what to do for the first three or four weeks afterwards. The general idea is to build up very gently and gradually the activities you can do for yourself, increasing not only your level of fitness to a modest degree, but also boosting your confidence. The confidence factor can be crucial, because being surrounded by hi-tech equipment and medical staff for several days can make you believe that you cannot survive without it.

At around four to six weeks the secondary prevention programme can begin in earnest. From now on the term 'heart patients' will include those who have had a heart attack, heart surgery or who have angina.

Boosting confidence is one good reason why all secondary prevention programmes should begin with a stress test. The

stress test is designed not to put you under stress,
but to see how much exercise you can do without becoming stressed. You will do the test on an exercise bicycle or treadmill linked to heart-monitoring equipment. An ECG tracing will help medical staff assess the state of your heart. They will also advise you of your safe heart rate. This is the rate which you should not exceed while exercising.

Everyone in the group will be taught how to take his or her pulse and calculate a safe heart rate. For people who are on drugs – particularly the beta-blockers which artifically slow your heart down – the safe heart rate will be calculated differently. Some people find taking their pulse and doing calculations very difficult. If this is the case, simply follow the same rules as non-heart patients and exercise to the point where you become slightly breathless. Always stop if you feel any pain.

The exercises should be aerobic (see chapter seven) and regular – two or three times a week for 20 or 30 minutes at a time.

These early exercise sessions will be supervised by someone with medical training because, in the unlikely event of a heart patient getting into difficulties, or even having a heart attack, a trained person will know the correct cardio-pulmonary resuscitation, or CPR, techniques and will be able to use a defibrillator if necessary.

One of the most important things that you will learn on a coronary prevention programme is that not only is it possible, but desirable, to exercise independently. This can be quite difficult to come to terms with, particularly if the programme is based on a hospital where the medical expertise is to hand. Some programmes get around this by deliberately basing the programme away from the hospital, in a health or leisure centre, for example. Being located in the community might also make the programme easier to get to. Many people live several miles away from a hospital and transport may be a problem.

But, wherever the programme is based, the ultimate aim is the same – to give you the skills and encouragement you need to make exercise a regular and permanent part of your life. The amount of exercise you do will depend on your particular circumstances. It is not unusual for heart patients to become fitter after a prevention programme than they have ever been in their lives.

Because of the dramatic improvement that some heart patients can achieve with exercise, many prevention programmes concentrate on this aspect. Most also include educational sessions. The information on smoking, diet and stress will be the same as that described in earlier chapters, but you may have the added benefit of discussing the issues with the experts – dietitians, physiotherapists and counsellors who may be based in the hospital or who can visit the programme.

Sex

Even at the best of times sex is a subject which many people find difficult to discuss, and following a heart attack or heart surgery is not the best of times. Angina sufferers too may worry that having sex will bring on an attack. The most often quoted guideline as to whether or not you are ready to resume sexual relations is that if you can climb two flights of stairs without pain or breathlessness, then you will be OK. Stair-climbing is really a rough guide to how fit you are feeling. Any other rough guide – walking down the road and back, doing some of the exercises you learnt in the programme – will do just as well. The most important thing is not to worry, as this will increase your stress level and increase the risk of an angina attack.

Talk to your doctor if you need reassurance about your level of fitness. He or she may prescribe drugs, such as nitrates, which will help to prevent an angina attack brought on by exertion such as sex. Remember that your doctor has come across much more embarrassing problems than yours.

If you really cannot face your doctor, go to a counsellor – your doctor may even refer you to one. Relate (formerly the Marriage Guidance Council) should also be able to help. The important thing is to do something. The problem will not go away if you ignore it and the longer you leave a sexual problem, the more likely it is to cause tension between you and your partner – the last thing you need at this stage in your life.

Driving

Driving is another activity which most patients are keen to get back to. Generally speaking most heart patients will be able to drive their car again provided they have made a good recovery or their angina is well controlled. You must, however, inform DVLC, and your insurance company too.

Getting back to driving is a mixed blessing because it may remove one of the key incentives to exercise – lack of motor transport. Once you are mobile, you will obviously want to get around but, unless long distances are involved, it would be better to walk or even cycle if your fitness level will allow it. Driving not only gives you no exercise but can also increase your stress level – a double disadvantage.

Being unable to drive is a much more serious problem if, before your coronary problem, you drove for a living. Very rarely, if your heart attack was very minor and tests show that you have made a full recovery, an exception may be made. In general, though, you will not be able to hold a Heavy Goods Vehicle (HGV) licence or a Public Service Vehicle licence. The decision to ban someone from their livelihood is not taken lightly but the risk to the public is considered too great to allow heart patients to continue as professional drivers.

Back to work

Whether you were a driver or not, employment often looms large as a problem for heart patients. More often than not it is possible to return to work if you want to – to either exactly the same job or to a similar but less demanding one. How soon you get back to work depends on you, your employers and your doctor. Some doctors lean towards getting you back to normal as soon as possible, arguing that there is nothing like getting back into the swing of things to prove that you are not an invalid. Others say there is no rush. Taking time to take stock of your life and deciding to make changes – perhaps at work as well as at home – might be more important. After all, what is the point in racing back to the situation which might have contributed to your coronary heart disease in the first place?

If money is a problem getting back to work might be a necessity. Make sure that you have checked out all the benefits that you might be entitled to because this could buy you some time while you decide what to do. You might even decide that you can manage without going back to work. If you have been in hospital you can chat to the hospital social worker. The Citizens Advice Bureau is a good starting point.

Women and secondary prevention

There is some evidence that women fare rather badly out of secondary prevention programmes. Sometimes female heart patients simply are not offered a place on the programme. Even if they are, women tend to be poorer attenders. And even if they do attend, they seem not to improve as much as the men.

It is not really clear why this is so. To begin with, the prevention programmes may not offer the kind of advice that female heart patients want. One study, for example, found that female heart patients were given no information at all about resuming sexual relations.

Another difficulty might be that women may not get as much support from the family. Whereas male heart patients in some studies complained of being 'molly-coddled' when they got home by over-cautious relatives, female heart patients seemed to be ignored by insensitive husbands and children who expected normal household service to be resumed as soon as possible! The solution here is to involve the family in the prevention programme from the beginning.

Prevention for all the family

In fact there is some evidence that involving the whole family can improve the prospects for the heart patient, whether female or male. It makes sense that if your family looks at your exercise programme, they will have a more realistic idea of your fitness level – no molly-coddling and no leaving you to it either. They might be inspired to take up some exercise themselves! The same applies to the information and advice on smoking, diet and stress. It's much more sensible if each member of the family eats a healthier diet and reduces his or her coronary risk too, than for you to eat special food while they live off chips and cakes. If someone won't stop smoking, he or she might be persuaded not to smoke in the house because of the damaging effect on your health. And an appreciation by the whole family of the role of stress in coronary heart disease might make everyone's life a little more relaxed.

And remember that, if you have children, your heart attack immediately adds a risk factor to their own profiles.

Who benefits?

It's never too late to reduce your risk of coronary heart disease. Progress may not be smooth and you will have good days and bad days. But there's almost always some room for improvement.

The only problem with secondary prevention is that not everyone who would benefit from it gets the chance to take part. A survey in 1989 showed that only about a third of district health authorities in the country offered any kind of programme to people who had had a heart attack or heart surgery. The figures are not available for people with angina, but they are likely to be even lower. The Coronary Prevention Group keeps a list of hospital-based programmes which is available to any enquirer, but unless you are lucky or are prepared to travel some distance you probably will not be able to join a prevention programme. The Coronary Prevention Group is working with other organisations to try to encourage the development of secondary prevention programmes in the National Health Service. Our shared aim is for every District Health Authority to offer such a service.

Self-help groups

In the meantime, you could do worse than to join a self-help group of heart patients. Knowing that you are not alone with your problems can be immensely reassuring and, however good your doctor is, there is no substitute for talking to people who really know what it is like. As well as being a source of information, advice and support, self-help groups can sometimes develop into thriving social clubs, fund-raising organisations and even the secondary prevention programme that the area lacks. With the help of sympathetic local medical staff a self-help group can offer all the elements of a good secondary prevention programme, including the exercise sessions.

A formal prevention programme and a self-help group are not necessarily alternatives. In some areas people attend both, or move onto the self-help group when they have finished the formal programme. Unfortunately there are not enough self-help groups to go round. An organisation called Interheart (see the address on page 186) can provide a contact for your nearest group. However, you don't have to wait for your district health authority to act, you can always set up a self-help group yourself.

CHAPTER 10

SHARING THE LOAD – WHAT OTHERS CAN DO TO HELP REDUCE YOUR RISK

THIS BOOK has summarised a wide range of national and international scientific data about coronary heart disease. Although it is clear that scientists plainly don't know everything, a great deal is known about the factors which can increase the risk of developing the killer disease.

But there is no sense in reducing your risk of coronary heart disease if this leads to changes in your lifestyle which themselves carry a higher risk to health. So the question 'What are the risks if I change my habits?' has been carefully considered. The answer is clear. Giving up smoking, eating a healthier diet, becoming a fitter and more active person and learning how to deal with stress can reduce not only your coronary risk but also your chance of developing other diseases such as strokes and other circulatory diseases, chest diseases such as bronchitis, digestive disorders and some types of cancer.

If this way of living is so healthy, why isn't everyone turning to it? Surveys by the Health Education Authority's Look After Your Heart campaign show that although most people in the UK have a fairly good idea about what the risk factors are for coronary heart disease in general terms, they are sometimes confused about the details. Many people, for example, think that eating too much cholesterol is the main cause of raised levels of cholesterol in the blood, whereas in fact saturated fat is the main culprit. A common myth is that coronaries are the preserve of the high-powered businessman, but research has shown that the unemployed and the less well-off in general are more likely to die of a heart attack than businessmen.

Some of this apparent confusion about what health advice to follow may stem from contradictory messages about health that appear in the media. First you are told to eat less fat, then the newspapers claim you will be at risk from cancer if you do. Next you are told to exercise, then a magazine warns that you run the risk of dropping dead on the squash court. This book should help you to disentangle the web of claim and counter-claim in the media. The three key questions for any new stories you come across are:

- *How strong is the link?* Have several studies by researchers found a link between the new factor and coronary heart disease? If not, treat the new results with caution.
- *Is it a likely cause?* Does this new factor affect blood pressure, or blood cholesterol levels, or how the blood clots, for example? Or could it be just a coincidence?
- *What are the risks and benefits of changing your lifestyle?* In other words, would the inconvenience and/or difficulty of adapting your lifestyle to follow the new health advice, for example by cycling to work, be worth it in terms of the reduced risk of coronary heart disease?

Supposing that many people did manage to balance the pros and cons of changing to healthier habits, would they automatically make the changes? Not necessarily. What if healthier food were more expensive, or the local swimming pool were always closed by the time they got home from work? Many factors can make it more difficult for people to make the healthy choice.

This final chapter will look at the public policies which could remove those obstacles. The Government is an obvious linchpin in the public policy arena. The laws it makes, how they are enforced, the allocation of public expenditure and the level of taxes and subsidies are just a few of the ways in which Government can affect our behaviour for good or, literally, ill. And it is not just a matter of decisions at national level. Britain has been a member of the European Community (EC) since 1973 and, although the EC is not primarily concerned with health issues, its policies can none the less have a major effect on an individual's chance of developing coronary heart disease.

Industry and commerce also have a vital role in preventing coronary heart disease, both through their marketing and advertising practices and as employers concerned for the health of their workforce. Professional bodies, too, can encourage their members' interest in prevention. And the National Health Service is beginning to develop plans to prevent coronary heart disease.

This section will not list all the policies which could be introduced but it will look at the major policy changes which have been suggested to help reduce each of the main risks for coronary heart disease.

Smoking

The tobacco industry is obviously no supporter of the campaign to reduce the risk of coronary heart disease and of many other fatal and disabling illnesses. In the face of substantial evidence it continues to deny that smoking is a lethal addiction and uses its considerable powers to try to block policies which would help to discourage smoking, such as higher taxation, a total ban on advertising and the creation of more smoke-free public places.

Tobacco taxes

Increasing tobacco taxation has been shown (by Joy Townsend of the Medical Research Council's Epidemiology Research Unit, Northwick Park Hospital, Middlesex) to be highly effective in reducing the number of cigarettes people smoke. Although studies vary in their estimates of the size of the effect, they all show that if you increase the price of tobacco you decrease consumption.

It has been estimated that for every 10 per cent increase in price, there is a 5 per cent fall in the number of cigarettes smoked. This is not a permanent fall. For those people who simply cut down, rather than stop, it is important to keep on increasing the price every year, because if it is allowed to fall, apparently or in real terms, consumption will creep back up. Studies from the USA show that price increases have the greatest effect on stopping young people from smoking.

Some Budgets have increased tobacco taxes above the rate of inflation, which has helped to keep the smoking trend moving downwards. However, in some years there has been no price rise and in others the increase has been less than the rate of inflation, so the real price of cigarettes has fallen.

People have argued that the Government makes too much money out of tobacco taxes to be serious about wanting people to stop. But although the revenue from tobacco tax will go down eventually – i.e. when only a handful of smokers are left – in the short term tobacco revenue increases when taxes are raised. Meanwhile, putting tobacco prices up increases inflation. While no one wishes to fuel inflation, it may still be argued that health deserves a higher priority.

Tobacco advertising and promotion

Another area where health organisations and Government disagree is over the advertising and promotion of tobacco. The industry loses 300 customers each day to the undertaker, so to stay in business it has to find new customers. The tobacco industry relies on advertising to promote its products and naturally it focuses on the sector of the population which is most likely to yield new customers. The vast majority of smokers become addicted before they are 18. Once a person has become a smoker he or she stands a one-in-four chance of dying from the addiction.

In 1990 the Government's Health Education Authority spent £3 million to try to persuade people not to start smoking and to help smokers to stop. Books, magazines, newspapers and TV programmes often warn of the health risks attached to smoking, but all of this is dwarfed by the £100 million which the tobacco industry is estimated (by the Health Education Authority and Action on Smoking and Health) to spend each year on advertising and promoting its products. Its billboards flank major roads, its brand names appear on racing cars, its trophies are handed out to snooker and cricket stars and even the arts benefit from the wealth of tobacco companies.

One solution to this unequal contest might be to ban all tobacco advertising and promotion. A number of countries have done precisely that. Portugal, Italy, Norway, Iceland, Finland, Canada and Nigeria already have a ban and are soon to be joined by France and Spain. The question is: Do bans work? To find out, research was commissioned by the New Zealand Government. Thirty-three countries were studied during the years 1970 to 1986. This major investigation revealed a strong link between bans on tobacco advertising and a fall in tobacco consumption. Even if the tobacco industry does not actually set out to recruit new smokers with its advertising, the effect of making its brands look glamorous and exciting is none the less to encourage people – particularly young people – to smoke.

Another ploy by the tobacco industry to defend its promotional activities is to argue that consumers need to know about new and 'safer' cigarettes. However, the fact is that although low tar cigarettes may marginally reduce the risk of lung cancer, they do not reduce the risk of coronary heart disease. In fact, smokers tend to inhale more deeply and frequently when smoking low tar cigarettes, in order to maintain nicotine intake. This increases carbon monoxide intake and hence the coronary risk. And regarding the 'educational' purpose of low tar product promotion smokers have been changing to low tar cigarettes even in countries where there is a total ban on advertising, so advertising is not essential for encouraging a switch to lower tar brands.

Tobacco advertising has long since been banished from TV and radio in the UK, but a series of voluntary agreements between the Government and the tobacco industry allow a wide range of advertising and promotional activities to continue. These voluntary agreements include a number of restrictions. The results of the 1990 HEA report on BBC coverage of tobacco-sponsored sport and the 1991 report on tobacco advertisements in women's magazines by Dr Jacobson of ASH suggest that restrictions may not be tough enough. One, for example, only bans smoking advertisements on billboards that are near to schools.

In the UK, government after government has found it easier not to tackle the vested interests of the tobacco industry, the advertising agencies and publications and the sports concerns which have come to rely on tobacco money.

Smoke-free public places

For many years non-smokers have put up with the smell of cigarette smoke. There was often no choice. Smokers used to be more numerous than they are today and it was considered acceptable behaviour to smoke anywhere. Nowadays smokers are a shrinking minority.

It has now been established that breathing in other people's cigarette smoke (passive smoking) increases the risk of lung cancer in non-smokers. The non-smoking majority are now demanding their right to breathe fresh air. A number of public and private companies are responding to these demands and are either banning smoking from their premises altogether or offering smoke-free areas to their customers. Planes, boats and trains have been in the vanguard of providing smoke-free areas for passengers. The increased risk of fire caused by smouldering cigarette ends has led to a total ban on smoking in London's Underground system. On many buses, too, only a few seats are reserved for smokers and smoking is now banned entirely on London buses. Restaurants, cinemas, hotels, leisure centres and even some pubs now provide smoke-free areas and the list is growing every day. People working in factories, offices and shops all over the UK are demanding their right to a smoke-free working environment.

Surveys by the Department of Health, the Health Education Authority, Action on Smoking and Health and Eurobarometer have shown overwhelming public support for smoke-free public places. Now that passive smoking has been proved by the Froggatt report, as well as by the US Surgeon General, the Medical Research Council in Australia and others to be dangerous to non-smokers, there is a clear duty on governments to protect the health of the majority from the habit of the minority.

Even the majority of smokers support restrictions on smoking in public places because, they argue, it means they smoke less, and, since many smokers want to give up, restrictions are an added incentive. The tobacco industry, on the other hand, denies that there is any health risk to smoking, whether active or passive. It argues that smokers are being persecuted and denied their right to smoke. In the meantime, it is up to consumers to claim back the right to smoke-free air.

The economic case

The UK used to be in the vanguard of tobacco control policies. In recent years, however, it has been overtaken by other countries which have introduced higher tobacco taxes, stricter advertising bans and legally enforceable smoke-free areas. The reasons for the UK's declining performance are not clear but cynics argue that the economic benefits of smoking are so great that the Government simply dare not tackle the smoking problem properly. The tobacco industry creates jobs, tax revenue and export earnings. The consumers of its products are more likely to die at an early age than non-smokers, which saves on pensions and other welfare costs.

Other experts have argued the reverse. Smoking, they say, costs industry a fortune in days lost through sickness, higher cleaning bills and greater fire risks. Smokers also cost the National Health Service money because they are often ill for long periods and need to be offered treatment and care.

So there are economic arguments on both sides, but only one argument for the government that cares about good health.

A healthy diet

There are hundreds, if not thousands, of possible elements in a healthy (or unhealthy) diet, and an enormous range of eating situations. How can healthy choices be encouraged?

Food labelling and advertising

Many surveys show that although people want comprehensive, consistent and clear information about the nutritional content of the food they buy, the information comes in almost as many forms as food itself.

In 1986 the Government introduced a set of voluntary guidelines which manufacturers were invited to use if they were intending to provide nutritional information on their products.

It was an attempt to create some order out of the chaos of nutritional labelling. At that time many products carried no such information and those which did could not be compared because most of the formats were different. Consumers' Association, the Coronary Prevention Group and many other organisations argued that voluntary guidelines would not work. Manufacturers would still be able to get away with giving consumers no information on nutrition and the guidelines suggested so many different formats that shoppers would still not be able to compare one label with another. Only food manufacturers who thought they had a strong 'selling point' in terms of the product's claims to promoting good health would introduce nutritional labelling.

Some five years on health and consumer groups have been proved right. A recent Consumers' Association survey showed that a quarter of products still carried no nutritional information at all and a mere 3 per cent gave all the information consumers need to be able to choose a healthy diet. There is little prospect of this situation improving in the near future. Despite the fact that the UK voluntary system has been proved worthless, the European Community agreed in 1990 to introduce a similar voluntary system. The only advantage of the EC system is that there will be only three possible variations in format – a full label, half a label or nothing.

But even the full label is insufficient on its own. Nutritional labels are often printed in very small type and use technical language. No wonder hardly anyone understands them. Contrast the dull lists of numbers with the bold, bright flashes on the fronts of packets and in advertisements: 'lowest in fat', 'high in fibre', 'no added salt', '20 per cent less sugar'. Recently, more ambitious claims about what the food can do have been evident, such as 'helps lower cholesterol'.

Unfortunately these claims are not helpful to the consumer. Two packets, both bearing the legend 'low fat', can legally contain completely different amounts of fat. The same is true for many other nutrients. Manufacturers do not even have to back up their claims with nutritional information; they can flash 'no added sugar' on the front and not mention the sugar content in the nutritional information on the back of the packet. A recent survey by the Coronary Prevention Group has revealed that this practice is widespread. Many claims are also selective, highlighting the 'good' nutrients and concealing the 'bad'. Breakfast cereals, for instance, often claim to be high in fibre, but hide the amount of sugar they contain by listing a total carbohydrate figure. Once again, these claims are controlled by voluntary guidelines, issued by the Government. And what about products which claim to lower cholesterol levels and imply that they can reduce coronary risk? The Coronary Prevention Group believes that some of these claims are misleading and possibly illegal. No food on its own can prevent coronary heart disease, besides which coronary risk always depends on more than one factor. If food manufacturers are going to spread the message about diet and health, then these messages must be balanced, comprehensive and clear.

The Coronary Prevention Group, Consumers' Association and others are campaigning hard for clear and useful nutritional information on every food packet, together with tough rules to govern claims in advertising and on packets. If you think a label or an advertisement is misleading, write to the Advertising Standards Authority or the Independent Television Commission (addresses on page 188). The battle will not be easily won: laws on food labelling and advertising are enforced by local authority trading standards officers or environmental health officers, who have vastly more limited resources than teams of lawyers from large food conglomerates.

But it is not just printed information that can cause a problem for hard-pressed local enforcement officers. About 90 per cent of the money spent on advertising food and soft drinks goes on TV adverts: £550 million every year. A recent survey by *Food Magazine* revealed that over half the advertising during children's TV was for food and soft drinks and that most of the products were high in fat, sugar or salt.

Although you will rarely see TV advertisements for potatoes, you will often see them for potato crisps, on which the profit margin is so much greater. About 60 per cent of the calories in a bag of average crisps comes from fat and, unless they come with a separate bag of salt, they are very salty. Most of the fibre and vitamin C in which the potato is naturally high has been lost in the processing. In 1991 a kilo (a couple of pounds) of potatoes would cost about 30p but a kilo of potato crisps would work out at about £6. The difference between potatoes and potato crisps (apart from the fact that the latter have a far lower nutritional value than the former) is that crisps have been processed. At each point in the processing stage – grading, peeling, slicing, blanching, frying, salting, packaging and packing etc. – a little more is added on to the price to cover the costs of the process and allow the processor to take a higher profit. That is why crisps are more expensive than potatoes.

The problem is that most food is at its nutritional best when it's closest to its fresh state. The more that food is processed, the more nutritional value it tends to lose. Many other foods meet the same fate as the potato – from oranges to marmalade, from chicken breast to breadcrumbed nuggets, from roast beef to meat pies.

Fresh raw products – fruit, vegetables, bread, fish and meat – tend not to have nutritional labels. These foods usually have a short shelf life and, in any case, fresh foods are less likely to have hidden ingredients that need labelling. But because producers are aware of the interest in nutrition, some are banding together to provide nutritional information leaflets about their fresh, raw goods. This is welcome news, but it is the information for processed foods that deserves the most urgent attention.

Catering

There is one area of healthy eating where you might feel you do not need to worry about labels and advertisements – eating out. You do not have to shop for the ingredients or cook them, just choose and eat. In fact the attractions of eating out are proving so great that more and more of us are doing it. In 1977 only 13 per cent of our total food bills were for eating out but by 1987 this had grown to 24 per cent – a massive total of £17 billion in that year and still rising. This works out at three or four meals a week each.

You might protest that you do not eat out anything like as often as that, but remember that this figure does not just represent restaurants, it includes fast-food take-away outlets, hotels, canteens, school meals, hospital catering and many more.

The Government's National Food Survey, which has been going on for 50 years and publishes its results every three months, is showing quite encouraging trends in the pattern of what people eat at home. We are eating more wholemeal bread, more low-fat milk, more fruit juices and so on. But the survey does *not* include food eaten outside the home. The figures we have for this sector aren't as good but they seem to show that we're taking the healthy eating message home – and leaving it there! Outside we're eating chips, burgers, sweets, fizzy drinks and all sorts of low fibre foods which are high in fat, salt and sugar. Eating these items three or four times a week, week in, week out, can have an important effect on your diet and there are some signs that the effect may be unhealthy.

There are several things the Government could do to help people choose more healthily when eating out. To begin with, it could lead by example. If you were to add up all the canteens in central and local government offices, school meals, hospital food, meals on wheels, armed forces catering, prison food, meals in old people's homes, food in state-run nursery schools and so on – you would soon realise that the Government is the largest caterer in the UK. Nutritional standards have been developed by a number of these catering outlets.

In fact, one public sector catering outlet at one time provided food that had to conform to nutritional standards: school meals. The Coronary Prevention Group and others have asked several times for these standards to be updated and reintroduced but our appeals have fallen on stony ground. This is more worrying in the light of the Department of Health survey, 'Diets of British Schoolchildren', which showed that children's diets contain a high proportion of fatty, low-fibre foods, such as chips, burgers and sweets.

Many school caterers (and other caterers in the public sector such as hospitals and the armed forces) have anyway taken the initiative and developed healthier standards. The results so far have been encouraging – more children are provided with healthy school meals, but the school initiatives that provide these meals tend to be isolated good examples, while other school meals services struggle on low budgets and falling customer numbers.

Perhaps private catering could also be improved. Many private caterers, for example in hotels and restaurant chains, have already started to offer healthy options on their menus. Improved training for catering staff might also help raise standards. Clearly it would be impossible to impose nutritional standards on such a diverse sector but the Government could make standard catering operations, such as fast food outlets, introduce menu labelling systems. For fast-food chains with a standard product it would be very easy to provide customers with information about saturated fat, fibre, salt and sugar content.

The food supply

One of the most important factors shaping what you eat is the food sector that the majority of British people rarely see – farming. Today it is not just what British farmers do that affects our food, but also what happens in the European Community's Common Agricultural Policy.

The CAP is a network of policies which has been developed over many years. These policies have been designed to support farmers, protect rural development and provide sufficient quantities of food for Europe's citizens. It can be argued that the CAP has not been particularly successful in achieving these goals but they are, at least, central issues in the policy-making process. The healthiness of the food supply, however, is *not* an issue which concerns Agriculture Ministers from EC countries when they meet to discuss the CAP.

The complexity of the CAP makes it extremely difficult to work out whether the CAP has been good for coronary heart disease prevention or not. Take butter, for example. It is high in saturated fat, so one way to reduce the saturated fat in your diet would be to eat less of it. The CAP has actually kept the price of butter quite high and this may have contributed to the fact that we *are* eating less butter. Unfortunately, even though demand for butter has been falling, farmers are still producing nearly as much of it – leading to the famous 'butter mountains'. One of the ways EC officials have developed to shift the supplies of butter is to sell it cheaply to manufacturers of cakes, biscuits and ice-cream. This keeps prices of these products down and consumption up, so consumers end up eating some of the butter.

This subsidised butter scheme cost the EC £77 million in 1990, which will eventually end up in all our tax bills. So even though consumers have chosen not to buy butter, we might still end up paying for it and eating it. On top of that, in 1990 the EC launched a £3.6 million campaign to persuade us to eat more dairy products, including butter.

A trifling £¼ million will be spent on promoting fresh fruit and vegetables, whilst fruit and vegetable stocks are destroyed to keep the price up. Contrast this with the £850 million spent in 1990 on CAP subsidies for tobacco. In response to such absurdities of the CAP, political pressure has been building up from several member countries to make changes. Some reforms have been made and more have been suggested but one thing is certain – the effects of the CAP on coronary heart disease will not feature in the negotiations.

While it seems to be perfectly acceptable to develop taxes, subsidies, quotas and all manner of mechanisms to defend the livelihood of farmers, promote rural development and protect the environment – all worthwhile goals – governments say it is not acceptable to use these mechanisms to prevent coronary heart disease. The Coronary Prevention Group disagrees.

To sum up, government, agriculture and industry could do a lot to make it easier for people to choose healthy food. Labels could be better, standards could be tougher and the CAP could put health high on its agenda. The Coronary Prevention Group and a whole range of other organisations are working on your behalf to try to make these policy changes happen.

Exercise

Human bodies are designed to be active. The development of coronary heart disease is just one of the risks you run if you don't exercise. Until relatively recently many people worked in agriculture doing hard, physical jobs, while others did demanding work in industrial settings. Housework was likewise an energetic occupation without many of today's labour-saving devices. Few people owned cars, so getting about was a case of cycling or walking.

After the Second World War the pace of change quickened. Agriculture became mechanised, new technologies were brought to industry and office work boomed. Vacuum cleaners and washing machines took the effort (if not the time) out of housework and car ownership rocketed. It has become normal to have an inactive life. If you feel exhausted some days, fatigue is more likely to be mental than physical because you're not used to physical activity.

However, cycling in towns and cities can be a dangerous business. Inhaling exhaust fumes is a health hazard and every year hundreds of cyclists come off worse in clashes with cars. Even walking can be dangerous if you live in an unsafe area. Often parents worry about the safety of their children outside the home, even during daylight hours and in some areas it's rare to see children playing outside unsupervised. Many children don't even walk or cycle to school. One survey showed that in 1971 around 80 per cent of children got to school under their own steam but by 1990 this figure had plummeted to 10 per cent.

No wonder that the bad exercise habits we noted in adults in chapter seven are affecting children, too. Research at Exeter University has confirmed this trend, revealing that most children have few activities which regularly raise their heart rates and exercise their muscles. The evidence presented in chapter seven indicates significant health benefits from increased activity, so the main focus of public policy towards exercise needs to be both on exercise as a means of transport and on special exercise and leisure activities. Southampton, for example, is pioneering safe cycleways through and around the busy city centre. Other councils could be encouraged to do the same. Good lighting and visible policing, for example, would help people feel safer at night to walk and to use public transport.

Much more could be done to make sure that the exercise facilities that already exist are fully utilised at educational institutions: colleges, universities and polytechnics as well as schools, have playing fields, tennis courts, swimming pools.

And it's not just the Government which could help. Many private firms have sports facilities which are not used as much as they could be. Even smaller firms, which don't have the money to construct special facilities, could at least install a shower at work. People who cycle to work in the mornings, employees who jog at lunchtime and those who have exercise classes nearby in the evenings would all find it helpful to freshen up before settling down to work or returning home.

Despite the 1980s boom in fitness and sports activities of all kinds (fun-runs, gymnasiums, aerobics classes, marathons and cycling) those people who have the highest rates of coronary heart disease and so have the most to gain from these activities – people on low incomes – are the least likely to participate.

Perhaps the National Fitness Survey will provide a much needed boost to exercise promotion policies in the UK. This survey started in 1990 and is a unique collaboration between the Government and industry to try to discover exactly how fit (or unfit) the British people really are. The results may be depressing but they might spur Government and industry on to tackle some of the problems outlined in this chapter.

Health education

Whatever government or industry does, or fails to do, it is important that people understand coronary heart disease and what they can do about it.

About 8 per cent of children have already tried smoking by the age of nine. Health education in schools should begin at an early age and continue throughout the school career. As well as looking at the dangers of smoking, health education should also cover healthy eating, exercise and dealing with stress.

Unfortunately, health education is not a subject in the core curriculum, it is not a GCSE subject, and one of the courses where health education used to be taught – home economics – has disappeared from school timetables. Time allocated for physical education, too, is shrinking fast, with plans for a mere 5 per cent of curriculum time devoted to sports and games. The theory is that health education will now be a cross-curricular subject, with different elements being taught in a range of core subjects – smoking education during science lessons perhaps, healthy eating during design and technology lessons, and so on.

But it isn't just what goes on during teaching time that is important – the so-called 'hidden curriculum' is also critical. There is little point, for example, in warning children of the dangers of smoking if staff are seen smoking on school premises. Why teach children about healthy eating if the school meals service serves chips every day and the tuck shop sells crisps and sweets more cheaply than fruit?

Schools need time, money and commitment to be able to develop comprehensive and coherent health education policies but time and money are in short supply. One unfortunate consequence of the lack of funds in some schools is that, where health education materials are scarce, commercial interests have stepped into the breach. The Meat and Livestock Commission, the National Dairy Council, the National Peanut Education Council of America and the British Sugar Bureau are just some of the industries which provide educational materials free or at very low cost to schools. Although some of these resources have been praised by teachers and many are of excellent quality, others are barely disguised advertisements for products.

Of course, a teacher can always reject materials but, unless a qualified nutritionist, with the time to keep up with the scientific literature, he or she may not always spot commercial 'sleight of hand.' And is it right that even the best of these sponsored health education materials are used in schools? With even the most careful approach commercially sponsored materials may not provide the most balanced view of a subject.

If you have school-age children and are concerned about the quality of their health education, the best option open to you is to discuss it with the staff or governors.

What about those of you who are long past school age? England, Northern Ireland, Scotland and Wales each have government programmes aimed at improving the heart-health of the region. The scale and particular approach of each programme varies but they all work with employers, the media and, perhaps most important of all, the National Health Service.

Health checks

The most important part of the National Health Service for preventing coronary heart disease is the primary health care team at the doctor's surgery. Over a period of five years, about 90 per cent of the population will visit the doctor, so if GPs offer preventive services almost everyone should have access to these services. In April 1990 all GPs entered into a new contract with the Government which is intended to encourage doctors, and other members of the primary health care team, to undertake more preventive work. It is still early days to assess what form this prevention is taking and whether it is working.

Under the new contract, if you visit your doctor you will be asked about smoking, exercise and dietary habits, and you will be offered a blood pressure test, height and weight measurement and urine analysis. You will also be asked about any family members who have had a heart attack and about any possible symptoms of heart disease. From this information is should be possible to assess whether or not a cholesterol test is also necessary. Putting all the results together, your doctor should be able to assess your personal risk and offer advice and treatment accordingly.

The problem is that all of this takes time – a good deal longer than the five minutes a doctor can usually allocate to each patient – and some surveys show that a few doctors aren't very interested in preventing coronary heart disease. They have been trained to treat people who are ill and, some say, it is more than a full-time job to provide them with a good service, let alone to deal with people who seem perfectly healthy. And even doctors who are interested often lack the time to keep up with the latest scientific information about coronary heart disease or lack the knowledge and skills to give people advice rather than tablets.

But despite the fact that doctors already have to do a different job in difficult circumstances, and despite the rather disappointing reaction of some of the medical profession, many doctors are already taking action to prevent the people on their register becoming patients in their surgery. They need several things to help them do an even better job. First, they need information and training. It may be many years since they qualified and scientific research is, as we have seen, uncovering more and more details about coronary heart disease all the time.

Second, they need other staff in the practice who are also well-informed and trained. The doctor doesn't need to take everyone's blood pressure – the practice nurse can do that. The doctor doesn't have to give everyone advice on healthy eating – a dietitian or health visitor can help there. The receptionist, too, has an important role in making sure records are kept up to date, progress is monitored and people are regularly called back for check-ups if necessary. These are just a few examples of what the primary health care team can do.

All of this costs money, of course, and it is too soon to say whether the funds which the Government has promised for prevention are sufficient for the task ahead.

A British disease?

No country in the world has introduced *all* the policies which we have briefly described above. But some countries have done decidedly better than the UK in reducing deaths from coronary heart disease. Since 1968 the USA has seen a 53 per cent fall in coronary deaths among 35 to 74 year olds. The comparable figures for Australia are 48 per cent and for Finland, 27 per cent. All of these countries used to have a worse record for coronary heart disease than the UK. All of them are now doing much better. For the same age group and during the same period coronary deaths fell by only 12 per cent in England and Wales, 9 per cent in Scotland and a mere 7 per cent in Northern Ireland.

Why have these other countries been so successful? No one has the complete answer to this but some studies of the American success have calculated that just under half the lives have been saved as a result of improved surgical techniques and drugs. In other words, they haven't quite succeeded in preventing coronary heart disease but at least people aren't dying so early from it. But more than half of the improvement *is* thought to be due to a climate of prevention – lower smoking rates, healthier diets and more exercise.

Another way of looking at the figures is to ask why the UK has done so badly? A clue to our failure came in an official report in 1989 which revealed that while the health service spent some £500 million treating coronary heart disease, the Government allocated a paltry £10 million to try to prevent the problem. And what we have described in this chapter so far gives little cause for optimism. The problem for politicians of every hue is that the benefits of prevention are in the long term. It may take 20 or 30 years before significant declines in coronary death rates can be demonstrated. The results of the money spent now may come too late to be counted as votes of appreciation.

For researchers, too, prevention presents a problem. To find out what kind of preventive activities work best requires large-scale, long-term studies and these are, by their very nature, expensive. Because these studies are, in effect, experiments with human beings, they are very difficult to control and the results can be unpredictable and difficult to interpret. A great deal of scientific research is funded by drug companies who want to see whether their product works (not whether the need for the drug can be prevented in the first place).

A great deal of money is invested in keeping things they way they are. But changes can happen gradually. Changes *are* happening. Smoking rates are falling, diets are becoming healthier, regular exercise is increasingly common. Rates of coronary heart disease in the UK are declining slowly at least.

You can help to speed up these processes. You can start by making the changes we have described in this book. This will help to reduce *your* risk of developing coronary heart disease. You can also demand your rights as a consumer such as smoke-free air, better information about the food you eat, and safer towns to walk and cycle in. Finally, you could consider your duties as a citizen. Your elected representatives at local, national and European level are supposed to be concerned for your health and welfare. Let them know what they should be doing to improve our coronary record.

At the same time you might be pleased to know that organisations such as the Coronary Prevention Group are fighting on your behalf to prevent coronary heart disease.

GLOSSARY

Aerobic Describes the type of exercise in which the large muscles move rhythmically over a sustained period of time, allowing an increased supply of oxygen to reach the muscles. Used to be known as isotonic exercise

Anaerobic Describes the type of exercise which requires short, sharp bursts of power and does not allow enough extra oxygen to reach the muscles. Used to be known as isometric exercise

Angina pectoris A temporary, squeezing pain in the chest normally brought on by exertion or stress. It indicates that the coronary arteries cannot supply the heart muscle with enough oxygen. The pain may be quite mild or very severe but, once the exertion or stress ends, the pain will fade after a few minutes

Angiogram See cardiac catheterisation

Angioplasty See cardiac catheterisation

Anti-oxidants Naturally occurring chemicals in the body which can neutralise free radicals. Certain minerals and vitamins, e.g. vitamins A, C and E, are anti-oxidants

Arrhythmia Any variation from the normal rhythm of the heart (see also bradycardia and tachycardia)

Aortic valve One of the heart's four valves, it connects the left ventricle to the aorta (see diagram on page 20)

Aorta The main artery, which carries oxygen-rich blood from the heart to all the other arteries in the body (see diagram on page 20)

Arteriogram See cardiac catheterisation

Arterioles Small arteries that branch off from a larger artery

Arteriosclerosis Refers to the narrowing and hardening of the arteries caused by atherosclerosis

Atherosclerosis Is the process in which fatty deposits and plaques grow inside the arteries, making them narrower

176

Atrioventricular (AV) node Part of the heart's natural pacemaker mechanism. Electrical signals from the sinus node pass through this AV node before reaching the ventricles

Atrium One of the heart's two collecting chambers (see diagram on page 20)

Bradycardia The heart beats too slowly

Capillaries Tiny blood vessels that connect the ends of the arterioles to the beginnings of the veins. Capillaries deliver oxygen to body tissues and remove carbon monoxide

Carbon dioxide A waste product from the body, which is carried in the veins and exhaled from the lungs

Carbon monoxide A poisonous gas found in, for example, cigarettes and car exhaust fumes

Cardiac catheterisation A process in which a thin tube or catheter is inserted via an artery in the arm or leg and guided to the heart. A dye which shows up on an X-ray is injected so that the activity of the pumping chambers (an angiogram) or the arteries (an arteriogram) can be observed. It is also possible to widen a narrowed artery by attaching a balloon to the catheter and inflating it over the blockage. This technique is known as angioplasty

Cardiomyopathy A general term to describe a diseased heart muscle, often of no known cause

Cardio-pulmonary resuscitation (CPR) A technique combining mouth-to-mouth breathing and heart massage to help keep alive someone whose heart has stopped beating – a cardiac arrest

Cholesterol An essential part of all the cells in the body which is processed in the liver and used, for example, to make hormones. Too much cholesterol circulating in the blood increases the risk of developing coronary heart disease. A high level of saturated fat in the diet is the main cause of raised blood cholesterol levels. Cholesterol in food – mainly in shellfish, liver and egg yolks – only slightly increases blood cholesterol levels

Collaterals Small, new arteries which can bypass arteries blocked by atherosclerosis

Complex carbohydrates An important source of energy (calories) in the diet, often naturally combined with useful amounts of fibre

Congenital heart disease Covers a number of heart deformities present at birth, ranging from the minor to the fatal

Corneal arcus A white circle round the edge of the iris which, in young and middle-aged people, can indicate raised levels of cholesterol in the blood

Coronary arteries The arteries which provide the heart with its own supply of oxygen-rich blood

Coronary artery bypass graft (CABG) A surgical operation in which one end of a healthy blood vessel is sewn to the aorta and the other end is sewn to a coronary artery further down from any blockage, thus bypassing it

Coronary artery spasm A sudden temporary constriction of a coronary artery, restricting blood supply and causing pain

Coronary thrombosis Formation of a clot in a coronary artery, cutting off the blood supply to the heart muscle

Deep vein thrombosis Often a result of prolonged bed rest. A clot forms in the veins in the legs causing pain and swelling

Defibrillator A machine which 'shocks' the heart into beating regularly again

Diastole The pause between heart beats, i.e. when the heart muscles relax and blood flows into the heart from the veins

Diastolic pressure Blood pressure at its lowest point, i.e. when the heart is relaxing between beats. A normal resting diastolic pressure is usually between 60 and 90

Ectopic beats 'skipped' heart beats – sometimes known as extra systoles

Electrocardiograph (ECG) A machine for observing changes in the electrical activity of the heart muscles. The electrical signals are recorded as a trace on moving paper – an electrocardiogram

Embolism Blockage of an artery by a fragment carried in the bloodstream, e.g. a clot dislodged from elsewhere

Energy (calories) A calorie is the amount of heat needed to raise the temperature of one gram of water by one degree centigrade. The measurement is used to express the amount of energy released by food when it is 'burned' or used by the body

Epidemiology The study of patterns of disease in communities rather than in individuals

Extrinsic sugar Sugars extracted from plant cells. Extrinsic sugar is digested more quickly than in its naturally occurring intrinsic form (see intrinsic sugar)

Familial hyperlipidaemia (FH) A genetic tendency to have very high levels of fats (or lipids) in the blood and, consequently, a high risk of developing coronary heart disease

Fibre See insoluble fibre and soluble fibre

Fibrinogen A protein in the blood involved in the clotting process

Free radicals Chemicals which may, in large quantities or certain combinations, cause damage to body tissues, e.g. the artery lining. (See also anti-oxidants)

Heart attack Coronary thrombosis leading to myocardial infarct

Heart block Partial or complete failure of the heart's natural pacemaker, which may leave the ventricles pumping at a very low rate of 20 to 30 beats per minute

Heart failure A general term describing the failure of the heart muscle to maintain efficient blood circulation, leading to congested lungs or swelling in the limbs

Heart scanning A process in which the heart's activity is observed by injecting small amounts of radioactive material (an isotope) into the bloodstream. It is sometimes known by the name of the isotope used, e.g. a thallium scan

High blood pressure See hypertension

High density lipoproteins (HDLs) Particles of fat and protein in the blood which remove cholesterol from the body's cells. The 'good' cholesterol

Hypercholesterolaemia Raised levels of cholesterol in the blood

Hyperlipidaemia A general term describing raised levels of fatty substances, e.g. cholesterol, triglycerides, in the blood

Hypertension Persistently high blood pressure which may, if left untreated, lead to stroke and hypertensive heart disease as well as increasing the risk of coronary heart disease (see also systolic pressure and diastolic pressure)

Hypertensive heart disease Damage to the left ventricle due to hypertension which may lead to heart failure and arrhythmia

Incompetence Usually applies to valves in the heart that are unable to close properly (see also regurgitant)

Inferior vena cava The veins from the legs and the body join up to form this large vein leading to the right atrium of the heart (see diagram on page 20)

Insoluble fibre Often called roughage, this type of fibre cannot be digested. It increases the bulk of foods and eases its passage through the body

Intermittent claudication Very similar to angina, but the pain occurs in the legs rather than the chest. The cause is the same – inadequate blood supply to the muscles due to atherosclerosis – and the pain will fade after a few minutes' rest

Intrinsic sugar Sugars still contained within plant cells, such as whole fruit and vegetables

Ischaemic heart disease Another term to describe the lack of blood supply to the heart due to atherosclerosis in the coronary arteries

Lipids Fatty substances in the blood

Lipoproteins Particles of fat bound together with protein

Low density lipoproteins (LDLs) Particles of fat and protein in the blood which transport cholesterol to the body's cells. The 'bad' cholesterol

Mitral valve One of the heart's four valves. It connects the left atrium to the left ventricle (see diagram on page 20)

Monounsaturated Describes a type of fat found in the seed or fruit of certain plants and thought to be neutral in terms of coronary risk

Myocardium A muscle which forms the walls of the heart

Myocardial infarct(ion) Death of part of the heart muscle due to lack of blood supply. This is often the result of a coronary thrombosis. As with angina the pain of myocardial infarction can be mild or very intense. A myocardial infarct differs from an angina attack in that the pain does not fade after a few minutes' rest

Omega 3 A type of polyunsaturated fat mainly found in oily fish. Some studies show that this type of oil makes the blood less likely to clot, thus reducing coronary risk

Omega 6 A type of polyunsaturated fat found mainly in seeds or fruit. Some studies show that this type of fat can reduce blood cholesterol

Osteoporosis Thinning and weakening of the bones, particularly common in older women

Palpitations An awareness of the heart beat. Occasionally it may indicate problems with the heart's rhythm (see bradycardia, tachycardia and ectopic beats)

Peripheral arterial disease Atherosclerosis in the arteries in the limbs, most frequently the legs

Plaque A patch growing inside the artery composed of fatty substances such as cholesterol and harder materials such as calcium, making the patch more brittle

Polyunsaturated Describes a type of fat found in the seed or fruit of plants (see Omega 6) or found in oily fish (see Omega 3). Often called essential fats or oils because the body cannot make them so they must be supplied by the diet

Pulmonary artery Carries blood from the right ventricle to the lungs where carbon dioxide is exhaled

Pulmonary valve One of the heart's four valves, connecting the right ventricle to the pulmonary artery leading to the lungs

Pulmonary veins Veins carrying oxygen-rich blood from the lungs to the heart (see diagram on page 20)

Regurgitant A term applied to blood flowing back the wrong way through a heart valve (see also incompetence)

Rheumatic heart disease The result of which can damage the heart valves due to a reaction caused by a bacteria (streptococcus)

Septum A muscular wall separating the two sides of the heart

Saturated Describes a type of fat found mainly, but not exclusively, in foods of animal origin. Eating too much saturated fat can lead to raised levels of cholesterol in the blood and so increase coronary risk

Silent ischaemia A decrease in the supply of blood to the heart

Sinus node The heart's natural pacemaker. It is a group of cells in the right atrium of the heart, generating electrical signals to trigger each heart beat

Sodium chloride Common salt

Soluble fibre A type of fibre which can bind itself to substances containing cholesterol, so may help to reduce blood cholesterol levels. It is found in beans, fruits, leafy vegetables and oats

Sphygmomanometer An instrument for measuring blood pressure

Stenosis Narrowing of any tube or vessel in the body. Usually applied to valves in the heart, e.g. mitral stenosis

Stress test An electrocardiograph (ECG) taken while the person is exercising on a treadmill or stationary cycle

Superior vena cava The veins from the head and arms join up to form this large vein leading to the heart's right atrium (see page 20)

Systole The heart beat, i.e. when the heart muscles contract and push blood round the body

Systolic pressure Blood pressure at its highest point, i.e. when the heart beats

Tachycardia The heart beats too quickly

Tricuspid valve One of the heart's four valves, connecting the right atrium with the right ventricle (see diagram on page 20)

Triglycerides A type of fat implicated in the blood clotting process, thus high levels may increase the risk of coronary heart disease

Ventricle The heart's main pumping chamber (see page 20)

Ventricular fibrillation Rapid and unco-ordinated beating which leads to a cardiac arrest

Very low density lipoproteins (VLDLs) Particles of fat and protein in the blood which transport triglycerides

Xanthelasmas Small fatty patches on the eyelids which can indicate raised levels of blood cholesterol

Xanthomas Small fatty lumps on the tendons at the back of the ankles and wrists which can indicate raised levels of blood cholesterol

Appendix

The following summary covers epidemiological studies referred to in this book

British Regional Heart Study

Subjects   7,735 men aged 40 to 59 based in 24 towns in England, Scotland and Wales
Factors studied   All major risk factors
Results   This study began in 1978 and is still going on, with more results being collected. Early findings confirmed the importance of the major risk factors: raised blood cholesterol levels, high blood pressure and smoking

Civil Servants Study

Subjects   9,376 British male civil servants aged 45 to 64
Factors studied   All major risk factors, but particularly the effect of exercise habits
Results   The civil servants were studied from 1976 to 1985. Those who took part in vigorous activity at least twice a week had less than half the heart attacks of the other men, even after taking account of other major risk factors

Doll and Peto's British Doctors Study

Subjects   34,000 male British doctors
Factors studied   Smoking
Results   The doctors' smoking habits were studied from 1951 to 1971. The study helped to establish the link between smoking and lung cancer, other lung diseases, a variety of circulatory diseases and coronary heart disease. Deaths from coronary heart disease in doctors aged 45 or younger were 15 times greater than in non-smokers of the same age

Finnish Mental Hospitals

Subjects 700 men and 600 women aged 34 to 64
Factors studied Low saturated fat diet
Results The study began in the 1960s and the group following a low saturated fat diet for six years had fewer heart attacks than the controls, though the relative reduction in heart disease was smaller for women

Framingham, USA

Subjects Around 5,000 men and women
Factors studied All major risk factors
Results This study began in the late 1940s and continues today. As with the British Regional Heart Study, the results have confirmed the importance of the major risk factors

Los Angeles, USA

Subjects Male military veterans aged 54 to 88
Factors studied Low saturated fat diet
Results Eight years after the study began in 1959, there were fewer heart attacks in the group following a low saturated fat diet than in the control group

Multiple Risk Factor Intervention Trial, USA (MRFIT)

Subjects Around 13,000 men aged 35 to 37
Factors studied Diet, smoking and hypertension
Results During the 1970s, special advice and care was given to the experimental group of men, whilst the control group of men were referred to their own doctors for 'ordinary' treatment. After seven years, although coronary death rates fell slightly more in the experimental group than in the control group, the difference was not large. Men in the control group *and* the experimental group changed their diet, smoked less and reduced their blood pressure

North Karelia Project, Finland

Subjects 180,000 men and women sampled in 1972, 1977 and 1982

Factors studied All major risk factors

Results This project is still operating and a range of health promotion activities are being used. Early results showed coronary death rates fell faster in North Karelia than in the rest of Finland and that men fared better than women

Ancel Keys' Seven Countries Study

Subjects 16 groups of men (totalling 12,000) aged 40 to 59 years from seven countries; Finland, Greece, Italy, Japan, the Netherlands, the USA, Yugoslavia

Factors studied All major risk factors but particularly saturated fat and blood cholesterol

Results Information was obtained during 1957-1962, with further follow up five and ten years later. The results showed saturated fat consumption was strongly linked to blood cholesterol levels. Raised blood cholesterol levels, in turn, were shown to be related to high rates of coronary heart disease

Whitehall Study

Subjects 17, 530 male civil servants in London

Factors studied All major risk factors, but particularly employment status

Results Information was collected between 1967 and 1969 with a seven and a half year follow-up. Men in the lowest employment grades were three and a half times more likely to die from coronary heart disease than those in the highest employment grades, even after taking major risk factors into account

WHO European Collaborative Trial

Subjects 60,000 male employees in 80 factories in Belgium, Italy, Poland and the UK

Factors studied Diet, smoking, weight, exercise, hypertension

Results A variety of health education programmes were tried in each location in the late 1970s. After six years there was a reduction in coronary heart disease. The results were not as good in the UK and it has been suggested that this was due to a lower level of health education activity

ADDRESSES

The following is a list of those organisations that may be sources of further information. As many of these organisations are charitable, please include an s.a.e. with any enquiry you make. Consumers' Association and the Coronary Prevention Group can be contacted at the following addresses:

Consumers' Association
2 Marylebone Road, London NW1 4DX

Coronary Prevention Group
102 Gloucester Place, London W1H 3DA

Heart Disease

British Heart Foundation
14 Fitzhardinge Street, London W1H 4DH

Chest, Heart & Stroke Association
CHSA House, Whitecross Street, London EC1Y 8JJ

Family Heart Association
9 West Way, Botley, Oxford OX2 0JB

Interheart
The National Association of Self-help Groups for Cardiac Patients, Carers and Supporters, 60 Barry Road, Netherhall, Leicester LE15 1FB

The following are government funded campaigns for the four regions of the UK.

Look After Your Heart
Hamilton House, Mabledon Place, London WC1H 9TX

Change of Heart
The Beeches, 12 Hampton Manor Drive, Belfast BT7 3EN

Be All You Can Be
Woodburn House, Canaan Lane, Edinburgh EH10 4SG

Heartbeat Wales
Brunel House, Fitzalan Road, Cardiff CF2 1EB

Smoking

ASH (Action on Smoking and Health)
5–11 Mortimer Street, London W1N 7RH

QUIT (National Society of Non-Smokers)
102 Gloucester Place, London W1H 3DA

Exercise

The Sports Councils are funded by Government to promote sport and physical education in each UK region.

16 Upper Woburn Place, London WC1H 0QP

Upper Malone Road, Belfast BT9 5LA

Caledonia House, South Gyle, Edinburgh EH12 9DQ

Sophia Gardens, Cardiff CF1 9SW

Stress

Alexander Institute
16 Balderton Street, London W1Y 1TF

British Association for Counselling
37a Sheep Street, Rugby CV21 3BX

British Wheel of Yoga
1 Hamilton Place, Boston Road, Sleaford, Lincolnshire NG34 7ES

Centre for Autogenic Training
Positive Health Centre, 101 Harley Street, London W1N 1DF

Council for Complementary and Alternative Medicine and the Council for Acupuncture
Panther House, 38 Mount Pleasant, London WC1X 0AP

National Association of Citizens Advice Bureaux (also includes Debt Counselling Centres)
115–123 Pentonville Road, London N1 9LZ

Relate – Marriage Guidance
Herbert Gray College, Little Church Street, Rugby CV21 3AP

There is no central organisation for assertiveness training courses but your local adult education service may be able to help.

To complain about an advertisement on television or radio write to:

Independent Television Commission and Radio Authority
70 Brompton Road, London SW3 1EY

For any printed advertisement contact:

Advertising Standards Authority
Brook House, 2–16 Torrington Place, London WC1E 7HN

INDEX